THE BETTER SEX
THROUGH MINDFULNESS
WORKBOOK

The Better Sex through Mindfulness Workbook

A GUIDE TO CULTIVATING DESIRE

Lori A. Brotto, PhD

The Companion to the Critically Acclaimed
Better Sex through Mindfulness

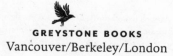

GREYSTONE BOOKS
Vancouver/Berkeley/London

To my brilliant students and research collaborators
who enabled the science behind the practice.

Greystone Books Ltd.
greystonebooks.com

Cataloguing data available from Library and Archives Canada
ISBN 978-1-77164-837-0 (pbk.)
ISBN 978-1-77164-838-7 (epub)

Editing by Nancy Flight
Copy editing by Lesley Cameron
Proofreading by Jennifer Stewart
Cover design by Jessica Sullivan and Fiona Siu
Text design by Fiona Siu
Cover illustration by Nayeli Jimenez
Printed and bound in Canada on FSC® certified paper at Friesens.
The FSC® label means that materials used for
the product have been responsibly sourced.

Rumi, J. "The Guest House." Translation by Coleman Barks.
A teaching story translated by Coleman Barks © by owner.
Provided at no charge for educational purposes.

Greystone Books thanks the Canada Council for the Arts,
the British Columbia Arts Council, the Province of British Columbia
through the Book Publishing Tax Credit, and the Government
of Canada for supporting our publishing activities.

Canadä

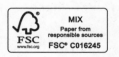

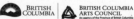

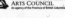

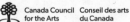

MIX
Paper from
responsible sources
FSC® C016245

BRITISH COLUMBIA

BRITISH COLUMBIA
ARTS COUNCIL
An agency of the Province of British Columbia

Canada Council   Conseil des arts
for the Arts   du Canada

Greystone Books gratefully acknowledges the xʷməθkʷəy̓əm (Musqueam),
Sḵwx̱wú7mesh (Squamish), and səl̓ílwətaʔɬ (Tsleil-Waututh) peoples on
whose land our Vancouver head office is located.

Contents

Foreword

WHEN A PATIENT who has concerns about low libido, or lack of desire, comes to see me, I discuss the inaccurate messaging about sex in our society and then explain that desire need not come before arousal but can follow it, that desire can be cultivated, and that a mindfulness program can improve sexual satisfaction and reduce feelings of sex-related distress. Almost always there is silence, followed by questions.

This information is typically new to patients, and it's a lot to take in, especially in the sterile environment of a doctor's office. Fortunately, there is a wonderful book that explains these concepts (and so much more) in a clear, approachable manner—*Better Sex through Mindfulness*, by Dr. Lori Brotto. It has been my go-to recommendation since it was published, and I prescribe it for concerns related to libido far more often than I prescribe pharmaceuticals. This book is revolutionary, and it is essential, especially in a world where pharmaceutical companies are eager to profit from distress and from misinformation about sex and desire.

But putting knowledge into action is hard for all of us, and that is why I am thrilled that Dr. Brotto has now written *The Better Sex through Mindfulness Workbook*. In this book, Dr. Brotto has converted her scientifically robust, in-person program into an essential step-by-step guide accessible to all. This workbook is for every woman struggling with issues related to desire, whether they are long-standing concerns unrelated to anything obvious or a new issue with a seemingly identifiable reason, such as stress or health challenges. Even women who are not facing issues with desire will find this workbook interesting and informative. I certainly did, and I talk about sex every day!

The practice of mindfulness may be unfamiliar to many, but Dr. Brotto's approachable language and style demystify the concept. She has anticipated the questions and the roadblocks that inevitably crop up, and the practices that she recommends are easy to do at home and can be incorporated into even the busiest of lives. And best of all, her recommendations are based on sound science.

I had long hoped that Dr. Brotto would write such a workbook. *The Better Sex through Mindfulness Workbook* is an evidence-based, practical, and accessible guide that is the perfect complement to *Better Sex through Mindfulness*. On a personal level, I am ecstatic that Dr. Brotto has provided me with another fantastic and much-needed resource for my patients. But the real win here is that every woman now has access to a guide that can help her put the science of mindfulness into practice and improve her satisfaction with sex.

Better sex is possible, and this workbook shows you how.

—DR. JEN GUNTER

Introduction

TOWARD THE END of my first book, *Better Sex through Mindfulness*, I noted: "Based on my own observation of mindfulness, I would argue that satisfying sex is quite simply *not possible* without mindfulness."

Now, four years later, I am even more convinced that this is true. Studies show that sexual difficulties remain high: up to 40 percent of women will experience loss of sexual desire, reduced pleasure with sex, struggles with reaching orgasm, or sexual pain at some point in their life. And issues related to lack of adequate sex education, societal stereotypes of what constitutes healthy sexuality, and the perception that "everyone else is having lots of orgasm-infused sex except me" are even more common. Among the various sexual complaints, loss of or low sexual desire is the most common not only in women but also in men. At the time of this writing, two medications for treating low desire in women have been approved in the United States and Canada. However, not only have they had little real-life impact on the prevalence of sexual problems or on women's sexual desire, but also they are prescribed to only a very small subset of women who meet very strict eligibility criteria. That leaves most women who have medical health issues or significant psychological struggles, such as anxiety and depression, or who are in a troubled relationship or do not have the means to pay for these medications, without care.

Stress levels have been at an all-time high in the past several years, and have been exacerbated during the COVID-19 pandemic (ongoing at the time this book went to print). Millions of people lost their jobs within a month of COVID-19 being identified as a public health threat in North America. Many of those who shifted to working from home had to make monumental adjustments to create a workable space there. As children moved from in-class to virtual learning, parents also found themselves responsible for their children's education. Wait lists for appointments with mental health professionals rose drastically during the pandemic, and many people were unable to access the care they desperately needed.

Despite speculation in the media that couples would be having more sex with "all this time on their hands" because they were no longer commuting to work and social events and children's extracurricular activities had been canceled, the data from a 2021 study painted a very different picture. Rates of partnered sexual interactions decreased as pandemic control measures increased, likely because people felt significantly more stressed as a result of the social restrictions imposed as part of those measures. In fact, many people who work in the field are already predicting that the pandemic will have a lasting effect on sexual desire and sexual behavior.

As the months of the pandemic have worn on, mindfulness has emerged as a way to help people cope with the stress and to begin to live more in the moment. While the topic of this workbook is using mindfulness to experience a more fulfilling sex life, the skills it will help you cultivate will be useful in a broader sense as we adjust to a new normal in a post-pandemic world.

WHAT IS MINDFULNESS?

Mindfulness can mean different things to different people, and even experts in the field define it in slightly different ways. For many years the only consensus was that mindfulness is neither emptying the mind of thoughts or thinking absolutely nothing, nor actively trying to relax or obtain a deep state of peace.

In 2004, a group of mindfulness experts came together with the intention of using a consensus-based process to come up with a definition of mindfulness that could be used for research. They eventually agreed that mindfulness has two important parts: the self-regulation of attention on a person's immediate experience and bringing acceptance, curiosity, and openness to that attention. That is, mindfulness comprises *what* you do and then *how* you do it.

In his 1990 book *Full Catastrophe Living: Using the Wisdom of Your Body and Mind to Face Stress, Pain, and Illness*, Jon Kabat-Zinn explained mindfulness as nonjudgmental, present-centered awareness in which each thought, feeling, or sensation that arises in your attention is acknowledged and accepted as it is. This means that *what* you are doing (i.e., paying attention) is as important as *how* you are doing it (i.e., nonjudgmentally). Mindfulness involves bringing your attention to a particular target, such as your breath (or part of your body or a sound), and focusing on the sensations that arise as you are paying attention to it.

You use curiosity to move even closer to the individual sensations and recognize that sensations are fluid, continually changing and evolving. It is not enough to notice that the breath is "fast and tense" and move on. What does "fast" feel like? Where is the tension located? What happens to those sensations of "fast and tense" the longer you pay attention? Do other sensations arise besides "fast and tense"? Does your awareness of those sensations remain fixed on one location? Do the feelings spread out and radiate? Is there a quality of "liking" or "disliking" those fast and tense sensations? And do the "liking" and "disliking" feelings change?

Paying attention to a single area in this way is not boring and certainly not a static experience, because, as you just saw, sensations are constantly changing. Each mindfulness practice is unique and your observations can be totally different each time. In this way, we are always new to mindfulness. As Kabat-Zinn and other mindfulness teachers humbly state, "We are all beginners."

The second part of mindfulness relates to the *how*. When we pay attention, we are not berating ourselves for not paying close enough attention or for repeatedly getting distracted. Rather, we bring kindness and gentleness to our practice and to ourselves. I often use the analogy of a puppy, whose attention can wander from a sound to food to a passing dog and so on. We expect that puppy to be pulled in a multitude of directions, and we do not insult or argue with it but gently tug the leash to pull it back and use nonblaming language to instruct it to stay put.

So many of us chastise ourselves when we find it difficult to pay attention. "What is wrong with me? Why can't I do this? I knew when I failed that yoga class that my mind was incapable of staying put!" This is not the approach we want to take when we get distracted during mindfulness. Rather, we want to treat our minds the same way we would treat that puppy—perhaps by saying something like "It's okay, mind. I know you're curious and it's tempting to be pulled in so many directions. I understand. But for this practice we're going to stay right here. We're going to focus, together, on the breath or the body. And it's okay if you get pulled away again. I'll just gently guide you back."

If we could only express the same kindness to ourselves as we would toward a pet, I expect that a lot of the negativity and self-judgment that so many people carry would dissipate. Try to keep this in mind as you practice: *What* you are paying attention to is as important as *how* you are paying attention.

HOW DO WE KNOW THAT PRACTICING MINDFUL SEX WORKS?

Over the past several years, evidence supporting the effectiveness of mindfulness in addressing sexual concerns has continued to mount. We now have scientific data showing the benefit of eight weeks of mindfulness practice for women who have Sexual Interest/Arousal Disorder, a diagnosis given when distressing low sexual desire persists for at least six months (though most women with this disorder suffer from these symptoms for much longer).

As part of a study my research team and I conducted from 2015 until 2020 and published in 2021, 148 women attended eight weekly group sessions during which a facilitator guided them through various mindfulness exercises and then encouraged them to continue practicing the exercises at home each day between sessions. The facilitators also provided the women with information drawn from the latest scientific findings about the nature of sexual desire and the causes of sexual concerns.

The results of our research showed that eight weeks' participation in a group mindfulness program significantly improved the women's sexual desire and reduced their feelings of sex-related distress. The women reported feeling greater satisfaction with their relationship and a reduced tendency to ruminate over sexual concerns. Their sexual arousal also increased when they were shown erotic stimuli in a private laboratory environment compared to how they responded to the same stimuli at the beginning of the project. Furthermore, after their mindfulness training, the women had significantly more mind-body synchrony, or concordance—the degree to which the mind's sexual arousal and the body's physical response are in sync when a woman is exposed to erotic triggers. For many women, these two aspects of arousal are not in sync, and many experts believe that this might be a factor in women's difficulties with sexual arousal and desire. The finding that mindfulness increased the mind-body sexual arousal connection has enormous implications for the treatment of women who are dissatisfied with their sexual response.

More remarkable was the finding that the women maintained these gains in sexual desire a year later, and that they continued to practice mindfulness, even though they were no longer part of a formal and regular mindfulness group, because they wanted to reap its benefits in other areas of their lives. Compare this to the effects of many pharmacological treatments, which wear off when you stop using the medication.

HOW TO GET THE MOST FROM THIS WORKBOOK

Women face multiple barriers to getting their sexual health needs met. In particular, many women feel embarrassed to talk to their health-care providers about their sexual issues, and when they do, they might be met with dismissive comments such as "Maybe you're not attracted to your partner." Or "You're fifty-five and postmenopausal. You shouldn't expect to enjoy sex like you did when you were twenty-five." Or "Maybe you're too wound up. Have you tried having a glass of wine?" It will come as little surprise, then, to learn that most women with low desire do not talk to a health-care provider but instead suffer in silence. Many turn to the internet for solutions but are often uncertain about what is fact and what is fiction.

Since publishing *Better Sex through Mindfulness*, I have received countless emails from people around the world asking how they can sign up for one of our mindfulness groups. Unfortunately, the groups we run in our UBC Sexual Health Research Lab are available only to research participants. However, I'm excited to share that our research team has been developing an online version of our in-person mindfulness program, called eSense, which delivers the same mindfulness and sexuality education and therapy over eight modules at a self-directed pace. Users work through the online material, read and listen to the mindfulness recordings, and practice the suggested activities each day, all at their own pace. This kind of flexibility allows for differences in people's schedules, readiness, and willingness to take on a new program. We have tested eSense with a small group of women so far, and the results have been very promising. Women report that the combination of engaging visuals, downloadable meditation files, and accessible stories and explanations have given them valuable information and skills for improving their sexual health and low desire. At the time of writing, we had progressed to more in-depth testing with larger samples of women to determine just how well it works, and for whom. The preliminary results suggest that our mindful sex program can be feasibly delivered online, removing many of the barriers that prevent women from getting the care they need for their sexual health.

In the meantime, those barriers prompted me to write this workbook. In our in-person programs, experienced facilitators guide the sessions according to a comprehensive treatment manual that my colleagues and I developed. Each of the participants in those groups and in one-on-one sessions also receives weekly handouts to work through on their own. This workbook leads you through the same practices and introduces you to the same skills and information that we deliver in our face-to-face mindfulness program—but you won't need a professional facilitator, a group of other women to work alongside, or to arrive at a specific time each week and pay for parking! Consider this your own personal "mindful sex coach" and use it whenever works best for you. I hope you will feel as though you are being individually guided in this program. And although you will be working through the readings and exercises on your own, know that you are not alone. Your story and your experiences are shared by countless others. I want you to imagine a large group of others working through the program with you at the same time—sitting and practicing mindfulness together. I hope you will be able to sense one another's energy and derive comfort and support from one another.

If you are planning to work through this workbook in a way that mimics our in-person and online programs, you might want to devote about one week per chapter, starting with chapter 1. But don't move on to the next chapter until you feel you've really worked through the daily mindfulness and other exercises. You might work through the exercises more quickly than one chapter per week, or you might take two to three weeks for just one chapter. Take the time you need. This is about you.

I also want you to know that what awaits you on the other side of this program is new awareness, a new appreciation of your body, confidence, optimism, and sexual satisfaction. I want you to trust the science, which shows that mindfulness works to cultivate sexual desire. I want you to imagine the thousands of women and other people from all over the world who have participated in in-person mindful sex programs and who are encouraging you to set aside your doubts or skepticism and give this program a try. And I want more than anything for you to experience firsthand how different life can be if you pay attention intentionally, compassionately, and in the present.

You'll notice that not every chapter is organized in exactly the same way. That's because they reflect the way we organize our face-to-face sessions. Chapters 1–8 all include at least one formal fifteen- to thirty-minute mindfulness practice, which is described in detail and provides an opportunity to work on the mindfulness "muscle" and create the foundation for your practice. You can read the instructions and then do the mindfulness practice unguided. Or, you can read the instructions and then listen to an audio recording of the practice on my website, www. loribrotto.com. (Note that there is no audio for the Back-to-Back Sensing and the Mindful Listening formal exercises.) If you plan to listen to the audio recording of a practice instead of reading the instructions, turn off the notifications for incoming calls or messages on your electronic device.

After each formal mindfulness practice I have included an Inquiry section, which contains three main questions that cover the following points:

· What did you notice?
· How was observing and noticing (the object, your thoughts, your movements, etc.) in this way different from how you normally pay attention?
· How might this mindfulness practice be relevant to your sexuality?

Each of these questions contains a series of other questions to help you reflect on what came up during your formal mindfulness practice after the meditation has ended (and the audio recording, if you are using it, has stopped) and put your observations into words. It also gives you an opportunity to reflect on how mindfulness could be relevant to and helpful for your sexuality. Because you are working through this workbook on your own, those reflections will be mostly private. But try to imagine that I am speaking directly to you through these questions and that you are responding to me as if we were in the same room. This might feel strange at first, but I promise you, I've seen it work well with many people.

While the three main questions in the Inquiry cover similar points for each exercise (except formal exercise 14, which focuses on Sensate Focus and uses a different style of Inquiry), your answers might not be the same for each practice. Each practice will be influenced by your mood, energy, attention level, and a variety of other factors coming into play at that particular time. There are no right answers. This is an opportunity to become more aware of all sensations arising in the present moment and to reflect on your practice. In the first few practices, I suggest how long to spend on answering each of the three main Inquiry questions. Over time you can adjust the amount of time you spend on each question based on what is arising for you most prominently in that moment. For example, sometimes you might want to spend more time with Inquiry question one (asking about what sensations you noticed), and other times you might feel pulled to spend more time with question three (asking how that meditation is related to your sexuality). I also share some responses to the Inquiry questions from women who have participated in our group sessions in most chapters.

Because the Inquiry is a critical part of the mindfulness practice, and one of the key ways that you'll experience firsthand how mindfulness could be relevant to your sexuality, try to take the time to answer all three questions and to imagine that I'm listening.

Most chapters also include at least one informal mindfulness practice that doesn't require you to read a step-by-step guide or listen to an audio recording. These practices provide an opportunity to bring mindfulness into your regular daily activities. Chapters 1 to 8 end with a section called "Time to Practice," where I summarize the recommended formal and informal mindfulness exercises you might do over the next week or two. Those chapters have a section titled "Struggles and Strategies" that describes some of the difficulties you might encounter with the exercises and offers suggestions for how to address them. These sections are based on both the challenges experienced by the women who have taken part in our face-to-face groups over the past two decades and their own suggestions for how to address them. I encourage you to think of your own possible strategies and to write them in your journal.

In addition to the mindfulness practices, this workbook includes information about sex and sexual health that we cover in our in-person mindfulness groups. Sometimes a lack of accurate information about sexual health is behind sexual problems like low desire. For example, if you do not know the causes of sexual dysfunction, you might not see those factors at play in your own life and be able to address them to improve your sexual health. Topics such as (peri)menopause are also subject to misinformation or outright lack of information. Given that some women develop changes in their sexual desire and arousal and problems with sexual pain during perimenopause, it is imperative that women have access to good, scientifically sound information. The information here is based on current (2021) scientific evidence, so if you are reading this years from now, there might be more information about sexual health that was not available at the time of this writing.

BEFORE YOU BEGIN

MAKING TIME FOR MINDFULNESS

In order to benefit most from the exercises, you will need to determine if now is the right time to start this program. This means thinking about whether you can devote some time each and every day for the next several weeks to your personal mindfulness practice—both the daily formal practice and the informal practices that you'll bring into your daily activities. It also means making time to do the reflective work, which will happen after your longer meditation practices and takes a more formal form, guided by the questions I provide. Journaling or keeping a diary of your practices and your observations during the mindfulness exercises can be a key part of staying committed to the program. It can help you identify times of the day or the week that work better for your meditations and can provide the necessary encouragement over time as you see yourself deepening your ability to be present and nonjudgmental. It's helpful to periodically go back and read earlier entries as you progress through this workbook. No one but you needs to see the contents of your journal.

If you are adding the daily practices and time for reading, reflecting, and writing into your schedule, something else will need to move aside or be put on hold. What will that be?

ALL YOU NEED IS A QUIET(ISH) SPACE

In addition to motivation and commitment, all you need is a quiet space to practice the formal mindfulness exercises. You do not need a yoga mat, healing crystals, or an essential oil diffuser, and you do not have to be able to sit in lotus pose. If privacy is a challenge, you can do any of the meditations with your eyes closed anywhere really, even if other people are around. Many participants in our program have told me they use their (parked) car as their practice spot because it is the only place they have peace and quiet. But if there is noise around, that is okay too. Background talking and other noise even provides an opportunity for you to experience firsthand how you'll deal with distractions and intrusions when you are trying to pay attention.

If you are listening to the audio recordings that accompany this book (see www.loribrotto.com), you might find a headset to minimize background noise helpful. In the recordings, I mention sitting in a chair in an upright and dignified position. You can use any chair you like or even a sofa. I recommend that you sit upright as opposed to slouching with your head held up by the support from behind, as this might induce a feeling of sleepiness. Some people prefer to do the exercises while lying down, especially if they experience chronic pain that makes sitting for extended periods of time difficult. The only caveat about practicing mindfulness while lying down is that you might be more likely to drift off and fall asleep. Keeping your eyes open is one way to reduce the chances of this happening. Still others prefer to practice mindfulness while in a standing position. Some of the exercises in this book invite you to stand and stretch.

I have mentioned drifting off to sleep a few times now, so you might be wondering whether mindfulness is an effective way to deal with insomnia. It is! Racing thoughts can stop people from falling (or staying) asleep, and because mindfulness teaches us to let thoughts be rather than getting caught up in their meaning and content, it has been evaluated as quite effective for addressing sleep disturbances. So, if you find that you are dozing off during the practices, try moving your practice to a time when you feel most awake, perhaps in the morning, or try keeping your eyes open while you do your practice. You can use your journal to track whether (and how often) you fall asleep during mindfulness practices. Although dozing can create a wonderful, warm, cozy feeling, mindfulness is really about falling awake, not asleep!

MINDFUL SEX STARTS WITH NONSEXUAL MINDFULNESS

This workbook will introduce mindfulness to you in a way that will allow you to learn and practice the exercises at home on your own. If you have participated in a mindfulness program in the past—for example, mindfulness-based stress-reduction or mindfulness-based cognitive therapy—the first few practices will be familiar to you. They are designed to help you move into a regular—ideally daily—mindfulness practice. The exercises in the later chapters are designed to gradually move you toward integrating mindfulness into sexual activity.

WHAT IF I'M NEW TO MINDFULNESS?

Among the hundreds of women who have participated in our mindfulness groups at the University of British Columbia (UBC), many were completely new to mindfulness. They had never even heard the term or been exposed to anything remotely similar to mindfulness, such as yoga, tantra, or concentration training. Others were experienced meditation practitioners or even taught meditation to others. And we have had many, many participants who fell somewhere between these two groups. I have seen firsthand that both experienced and inexperienced meditators benefit from this approach to mindful sex.

WHAT IF I'VE NEVER DISCUSSED SEXUALITY WITH A HEALTH-CARE PROVIDER?

Many of our past mindful sex group participants had never spoken to a health-care provider about their sexual concerns. Others had (or at least had tried). However, given that most women who struggle with low desire do not feel that their primary health-care provider has been willing or able to address their sexual concerns, experience tells me that our mindful sex program was the first comprehensive treatment that they had received. Furthermore, many women did not receive solid, comprehensive sex education at school, so we always include basic information and education about sexual health and sexual response in the program to fill any gaps in information!

Bottom line: Whether you are brand new to mindfulness or not, and whether you have ever spoken to a health-care provider about your sexuality or not, you are in the right place. I am glad you are here.

WHAT IF I'M SKEPTICAL ABOUT MINDFULNESS?

Consider the following three questions and then rate yourself on the 0 to 10 scale below.

1. How much do you want to see improvements in your sex life (in sexual desire, sexual pleasure, arousal, satisfaction, etc.)?

0	1	2	3	4	5	6	7	8	9	10
Satisfied with my current sex life				I somewhat want to see improvements in my sex life				I desperately need to see improvements in my sex life		

2. How committed are you to working on improving your sex life?

0	1	2	3	4	5	6	7	8	9	10

Not committed
at all to working
on my sex life

Somewhat
committed to working
on my sex life

Fully committed
to working on
my sex life

3. How confident are you that mindfulness will be helpful in improving your sex life?

0	1	2	3	4	5	6	7	8	9	10

Not at all confident
that mindfulness will
improve my sex life

Somewhat confident
that mindfulness will
improve my sex life

Fully confident
that mindfulness will
improve my sex life

I am sure that many of you reading this workbook are doing so because your answer to the first question was at least a 7. You are unhappy, dissatisfied, or distressed about your current sex life. Perhaps you are longing for more sexual desire, or you struggle with feeling sexually aroused. Maybe orgasms have become more challenging, muted, or absent altogether. Maybe sex hurts. Or maybe it is just not pleasurable in the way it used to be. Your motivation to improve your sex life is a major factor in helping you complete this program. In addition, your commitment to "doing the work" is essential. While using this workbook will increase your understanding and provide you with critical information, it will not be sufficient in itself. You will need to make a commitment to yourself to put into the action the various skills you learn as you go along. Perhaps most challenging of all, you will need to put yourself at the top of your to-do list.

Motivation is not the same as conviction, though. You don't need to completely believe in the power of mindfulness to improve your sexuality. In other words, your answer to the third question can range from full confidence in this approach to your sexuality to no confidence in it whatsoever! In fact, it is fine, and even normal, and perhaps even beneficial, to have a degree of skepticism about whether mindfulness skills will "work" for you. (You'll see that the word "normal" comes up several times in this workbook. We're all different and we all have our own understanding of "normal," but in this workbook it simply means common, generally accepted, or standard. In other words, I use it when I want you to know that nothing is wrong.)

In our research we routinely ask women whether they believe that mindfulness skills will help them address their sexual (and/or genital pain) issues before they start our mindful sex groups. We typically find a large range in how strongly our participants expect that mindfulness will help them improve their sexuality. Some are fully skeptical and have come to the group as a last resort, after trying "everything else" that their doctor (and the internet) has suggested. They don't have a lot of confidence that mindfulness will help restore their sexual desire. Others believe that mindfulness is an extremely logical treatment option for addressing their sexual difficulty and have a high degree of confidence that mindfulness will "work" for them. They might even have incorporated mindfulness into their lives (for managing stress, for example) before starting our program. I always find it interesting that we do not find any differences in improvements in sexual health outcomes between these two groups: the skeptics and the believers. In other words, it is entirely fine if you do not think that mindfulness will be helpful for you. The important thing is that you're committed to at least trying.

DOES MY PARTNER NEED TO WORK THROUGH THESE EXERCISES? WHAT IF I DON'T HAVE A PARTNER?

Much of the research on low desire has focused on couples in long-term, established relationships. But while I expect that many of you reading this workbook will be in a long-term monogamous relationship, I also expect that some of you will be single or in another relationship configuration, such as a polyamorous relationship or an open relationship. Some of you might be single but have casual sex partners.

Our research participants over the years have been a diverse group of people who cannot fit into a single box. We have found no differences in how partnered and single participants improved in terms of their sexual desire and satisfaction after our mindfulness groups. So, while the exercises in chapter 8 need to be done with a partner, the others can be done alone. In addition, chapter 9 includes information for people who do not identify as women.

Let's get started.

1

How a Raisin Can Be All You Need for Mindful Sex

FORMAL EXERCISE 1:
MINDFUL EATING PRACTICE

THE OBJECT

The goal of this exercise is to experience a piece of food through the sensations you feel in your body, not through memories, feelings, or thoughts you might have about it in your mind. Mindful eating is often where I like to begin any mindful sex program because eating is something you already do in your life regularly, and many people have experienced mindless eating (eating without really paying attention to either the food or the process of eating it). Slowing down and eating mindfully can be a potent way of experiencing the benefits of mindfulness and, if you are doubtful or skeptical about the value of mindfulness, this practice might provide enough evidence to convince you to move to the next mindfulness exercise.

WHAT YOU WILL NEED

· A raisin or other piece of dried fruit, or a piece of chocolate, a slice of apple or banana, or any other fruit, if you prefer
· A chair, ideally high-back

- A quiet space (remember that no space will be totally silent, and that is okay!)
- Your journal

I will refer to your piece of food as an "object" in part because I suggest a variety of foods you can use for this practice but also because I want you to set aside any feelings, thoughts, or memories you have about the food you have chosen. I want you to interact with it as though you are seeing it for the first time. If we refer to it as a cookie, the word "cookie" might elicit certain feelings, such as "warm, baked goodies," "wonderful aroma in my kitchen," "my childhood snack," or "guilt."

This practice will take about ten minutes.

STEP-BY-STEP GUIDE TO MINDFUL EATING

- Sit on your chair with your feet flat on the floor. Keep your spine straight and head up.

- Let's start by examining the object. Place it on the palm of one hand and set your gaze upon it. With your eyes open, take a few deep breaths. What details can you observe?

- Describe the color to yourself. Become aware of the object's shape. Look at the details on its surface. Do you notice smooth or rough patches? What happens to the light reflecting off the surface when you move your palm around?

- Can you describe the texture? Are there peaks and valleys?

- How else would you describe the shape of the object to someone if you were seeing it for the first time?

- Close your eyes and sense the weight of the object in your palm. See if you can focus even more sharply on the feelings in your palm as you sense the object resting there.

· Observe it for a few more moments.

· You might get distracted by other sounds in the room. You might think to yourself, "How is looking at a piece of food relevant to my sexual desire?" You might even feel silly. If any of these or other thoughts or feelings come up, acknowledge that they are there and then set them aside and return your attention to sensing your object.

· Touch the object with a finger from your other hand. Is it rough or smooth? Soft or hard? Thick or thin? Heavy or light?

· Lift it to sit under one nostril and continue to breathe normally. What smells do you sense?

· Close your eyes and continue to breathe in the odor of the object. Is it different when your eyes are closed? Try to focus even more closely on the smells as you breathe a bit deeper and take in the aroma.

· Move the object to the other nostril and continue to breathe in, first with your eyes open and then with eyes closed.

· Now bring the object to one ear. It might not make any sound when it is just resting in your palm or held between your fingers. What happens when you move it around between your fingers? How would you describe the sound? Its volume, tone, pitch, duration? If it makes no sound, you can notice that too. What is it like to sense silence?

· Close your eyes for a moment and tune in to your body to take note of any new sensations that arise now as you are in silence.

· Bring the object to your lips, but don't place it inside your mouth. What sensations do you feel against your lips? Where is your attention now as you are sensing how it feels against your lips? Are you having thoughts such as "I want to eat this!"

or "I hope no one is watching me play with this piece of food!"? Having thoughts like these is common and nothing to worry about. Just take notice of them, then let them fade away into the background of your awareness as you return the focus of your attention to the sensations of the object against your lips.

- You might notice that you are starting to salivate. If you do, what does that feel like? Bring a friendly curiosity to the feelings of salivation. Don't interpret what the salivation means; rather, just sense it.

- Now place the object in your mouth. Pause and feel it. What sensations are most prominent for you? Where are those sensations located?

- Do you sense feelings in other parts of your body? Did you start chewing? If so, stop.

- Let the object just rest on your tongue without chewing. What sensations do you feel on your tongue? Is saliva starting to build? If so, what sound does it make? If not, that is fine too. There are no rules other than to pay attention.

- Now you can take one slow, deliberate bite. Move closer to the actual sensations. You can keep your eyes open, or close them, or alternate between the two. The object might start to slowly slide down your throat (your esophagus). If it does, what does that feel like?

- Take a few more slow, intentional chews and continue to observe the remnants of the object as it slides down your esophagus. Shift your attention slightly to your teeth and then your jaw. Observe what those parts of your body feel like in this moment.

- Most or all of the object has likely been consumed now. Do you notice any aftertaste?

- Focus even more closely on the individual sensations that make up the aftertaste. What are the subtle flavors?

- If there is no aftertaste, you can take note of what absence of sensations feels like.

- Finally, take a few moments to expand the reach of your awareness to your body as a whole. What part of your body attracts your attention? What sensations do you notice there?

- You may have thoughts about this exercise. Do not ignore them or challenge them. Continue to focus on physical sensations in your body. This means acknowledging any thoughts that are there and letting them be.

- Finally, take a few deep breaths before you move on to the Inquiry.

THE INQUIRY

If you were standing during this eating practice, you could sit down now. If you were sitting, you could change your position or posture. Try to spend the next ten to fifteen minutes reading, thinking about, and answering the following three questions. You can say your answers aloud, write them down in your journal, or simply reflect on them. Whichever option you choose, take the time to consider each question in detail.

QUESTION 1. What did you notice during this practice?

Consider what sensations arose during this practice. Focus on the "bare sensations" you noticed rather than interpreting the sensations or making inferences about what the practice means. By bare sensations, I mean sensory qualities of the object, such as its temperature, texture, vibrations, intensity, location, and so on. What other sensations were you aware of? Can you describe them in detail? How long did each sensation last? What else came up for you as you engaged with your object? How did you handle distractions? Did you sense an urge to chew, and if so, what did you do with that urge? Take time to think about each of these questions before moving on to question 2.

QUESTION 2. How was paying attention to your object, in the way you just did, different from how you normally interact with that object?

If you chose a raisin, for example, how was your experience of eating a single raisin this way different from how you usually consume raisins? Try to be as detailed as possible in describing how this experience was similar to or different from how you typically eat the food you chose. In what ways was it similar? In what ways was it different? What struck you the most? Take time to think about each of these questions before moving on to question 3.

QUESTION 3. How was this exercise relevant to your sexuality?

How was observing your piece of food in the way that you did relevant to your sexual desire or sexual arousal? How was the attention you harnessed during this exercise important for understanding your sexual response? What learnings can you take from this Mindful Eating exercise to apply to your sexual health? How can this practice of mindful eating be used to improve aspects of your sexual life? Remember that there is no single correct answer. Any observation you make is useful and important. You have now completed the Mindful Eating practice.

RESPONSES TO THE MINDFUL EATING PRACTICE
When we ask question 1 of the Inquiry in groups of women who use a raisin as their object in our in-person mindful sex groups, we invariably hear a variety of different responses. Here is a selection of responses we have heard in the past:

· I never realized just how many ridges a raisin has!

· The flavor of the raisin was so much more intense than when I remember eating raisins in my regular life.

· My mouth was full of saliva, and I never realized that I could salivate because of a piece of food that is just resting against my lips.

· I actually do not like raisins, but I noticed that my feelings of dislike were rather minimal because I was so intently focused on doing this exercise.

· I surprised myself by how much attention I could bring to this one little object!

When we ask the women question 2, about how eating the object in this way is different from how they normally eat it, there is a near universal response that they have never spent ten minutes eating a single raisin! Some find the exercise too slow and say that they felt impatient doing it. If this was your experience, impatience might be a theme elsewhere in your life. The most common response we receive to this question is:

· I never eat raisins this way! I usually grab a large handful and pop them all into my mouth at once, often swallowing without even chewing!

Sometimes a woman will comment that the surface of the raisin resembles a vulva! As interesting as that observation is, the intent of the exercise and any other formal mindfulness practice is not to elicit a sexual meaning but to simply observe sensations that arise, exactly as they are, setting aside expectations, judgments, and inferences.

When we ask women the third question, about how this exercise might be relevant to their sexual health, they make the link between mindfulness and sex themselves. Here are some responses we have heard in the past:

- When I was salivating, it made me think about anticipation. Maybe I was salivating because I was thinking about putting the food in my mouth but had not yet [done that]. Maybe if I just slowed down before sexual activity and paid attention, I might feel anticipation for it in the same way my mouth was anticipating eating the raisin by salivating.

- It taught me that slowing down can be very powerful for truly feeling.

- I was struck by how much more intense sensations are when I just pay attention. I wonder if sexual feelings might be stronger if I were more mindful.

- I noticed I was on "auto-pilot" while trying to sense the raisin. I wonder if I'm also on auto-pilot during sex. In other words, my body is going through the motions but my mind is elsewhere.

As you answer the third question you'll experience firsthand the relevance of mindfulness to your life and your sexuality. The connections you make between your mindful observations and your sexuality are far more powerful for solidifying these practices than me trying to convince you how and why they work. Seeing (and experiencing) is believing!

EDUCATION ABOUT SEX: DEFINITIONS

SEXUAL RESPONSE

After this eating meditation, you might have made a direct link between slowing down and feeling more sexual desire, or you might have realized that noticing sensations in your body can positively influence your sexual arousal. Both of these responses mean you're already connecting the mindfulness exercises to aspects of your own sexual response.

But what do we mean by "sexual response"? Can you define sexual desire? Can you differentiate desire from arousal from other parts of sexual pleasure? How would you know if you were sexually satisfied?

SEXUAL AROUSAL

Sexual arousal is a feeling that includes both mental and physical aspects of sexual excitement. Mentally, a woman might feel "turned on" or "awakened sexually." Physically, she might feel flushed and notice that her heart rate and breathing have quickened. She might feel warmth, tingling, dampness, or muscle contractions in her genitals. These feelings of sexual excitement might start in anticipation of sex or once some sexual touching or stimulation has begun.

Does this definition of arousal align with your definition? Sexual arousal can be very subtle, and some women are not aware that they are aroused unless they touch themselves and feel signs of arousal such as an increased heart rate, increased skin sensitivity, or vaginal wetness. There is no need to feel alarmed if you cannot sense your own arousal.

As we practice mindfulness skills together over the next several weeks and I guide you to pay attention to sensations in your body, you might notice signs of arousal at times. When you do, pay attention to those sensations, moving your attention even closer to their source, following them from start to finish, and tuning in to their intensity as well as fluctuations in intensity. For many women, sexual arousal is the first part of sexual response that they notice when they are engaging in sex, either with a partner or alone. Arousal jump-starts the full sexual response cycle and is the pathway to sexual desire.

A loss of sexual arousal might be what drew you to this workbook. Some women experience loss of arousal as not feeling sexually excited in their bodies. Perhaps the triggers that used to elicit their sexual arousal are less effective than before or no longer work at all. Some women experience a physical numbness in parts of their body when they are being touched.

Others experience a loss of vaginal lubrication that can cause discomfort or pain during penetration. Penetration by a penis, dildo, or finger might be impossible because it is too painful. If any of these resonate with you, you are in the right place. We will explore how paying attention, nonjudgmentally, moment by moment, might be useful for rekindling feelings of arousal.

SEXUAL DESIRE

Sexual desire can be even harder to define than sexual arousal, even though the term is commonly used to express an interest in sexual activity. It can be a clear feeling of lust, libido, sexual drive, or something more subtle—a wish, even a "decision," or a motivation or reason for sex. It can be experienced as a physical urge to engage in sex, or as a desire for more sexual stimulation once a sexual encounter has begun and you start to notice sexual arousal. Some of the signs that a woman feels sexual desire include initiating sex by herself or with her partner, being receptive to her partner's sexual initiation, thinking or fantasizing about sex, or being responsive during a sexual encounter.

Loss of desire can be experienced as no longer thinking about, initiating, craving, or being motivated to have sex. For some women this loss of desire is abrupt, and they can define a "before" and "after" point or event. For other women, the loss of desire is far more gradual, perhaps occurring over months or even years. Low or loss of desire is very common and can be a great source of distress.

SEXUAL PLEASURE

Sexual pleasure is another term people commonly use to refer to their sexual response. Sexual arousal and desire work together to make sex feel good. Pleasure can be experienced in the body (it feels good physically) or in the mind (it feels good emotionally). What makes sex pleasurable can differ from person to person and from encounter to encounter. When women in a 2016 research study were asked directly how they define sexual pleasure, solitary pleasure (pleasure you feel when sexual on your own), and dyadic pleasure (pleasure you feel when being sexual with another person), they offered different descriptions of each, albeit with some points of overlap. For example, the women in the study revealed that the autonomy of solitary sexual activity allows them to direct their own sexual fantasy, where and how to stimulate themselves, and the nuances of the activity. This autonomy can create an intense physical pleasure and also emotional feelings of freedom, self-reliance, and control. Partnered sexual activities, in contrast, might entail prioritizing a partner's pleasure, although partnered sex and giving a partner pleasure can also elicit feelings of empowerment and achievement and thus heighten feelings of emotional pleasure.

A loss of pleasure can be devastating. "Pleasure" can also be challenging to define and is more of an overall subjective feeling that might not be easy to measure. Most women who lose feelings of sexual pleasure do not seek help, usually because they do not see their concerns as worthy of professional attention or they fear being dismissed by a health-care provider.

ORGASM

Orgasm is often considered the climax of sexual pleasure. It typically involves a peak sensation of intense pleasure that creates a state of altered consciousness and feelings of well-being and contentment. Many women experience involuntary pelvic floor muscle contractions at the time of orgasm.

The importance women and their partners place on the woman's orgasm during sexual activity differs from relationship to relationship and even over the course of a single relationship. Most women experience orgasms from stimulation to the external genitals, such as the clitoris, and sometimes the breasts.

Vaginal penetration does not lead to orgasm for the majority of women, so not reaching orgasm during intercourse is not necessarily a sign that anything is wrong.

For women who have never experienced an orgasm, sex education, learning how to touch and stimulate yourself for pleasure, and mindfulness practices that teach you to be fully aware of the sensations in the moment and challenge the tendency to focus on the end goal are very important. Some women experience an abrupt change in their ability to experience orgasm, and in such cases, it is important to look at physical and medical contributors such as a surgery, a new medication, or a medical illness.

Being overly focused on the end goal can hinder a woman's ability to reach orgasm. Asking herself whether she is there yet or whether her partner will notice if it is taking too long can interfere with sexual arousal and make orgasm more difficult or block it altogether. This is yet another situation in which mindfulness skills, which improve the ability to remain present and not focused on whether the "finish line" has been crossed, can help women to experience better sexual health.

SEXUAL PAIN

Sexual pain is any pain experienced during sexual activity, and includes pain at the vaginal entrance or inside the pelvis or abdomen. Many women experience occasional instances of pain at the vulva or vagina for a variety of relatively benign reasons—for example, a yeast infection or insufficient lubrication before vaginal penetration. Changes in estrogen levels during the perimenopausal transition or postmenopause, or while breastfeeding, can also increase vaginal dryness, which in turn can elicit pain during sexual activity.

Sexual pain can affect a woman's sexual desire and arousal. If it persists, the woman should contact her family doctor or gynecologist to arrange an examination. Sexual pain might also signal that a woman has a new physical health problem or that an existing problem is flaring up. Persisting pain with sex that causes a person significant distress is a medical diagnosis known as Provoked Vestibulodynia. A diagnosis of Provoked Vestibulodynia is given when the woman experiences distressing pain when her vulva or vagina is touched in any way and other visible causes have been ruled out. This condition affects up to one in five women, and treatment is typically provided by a gynecologist with expertise in sexual medicine and vulvar health.

Our research team published a study in 2019 that found that women with Provoked Vestibulodynia who participated in group mindfulness exercises felt less intense pain immediately after the group sessions. When they were reassessed a year later, their pain was still less intense, their sexual function in general had improved, and their tendency to catastrophize, or imagine the worst (e.g., my pain will never end), about the pain had decreased. If you experience pain with sex, the mindfulness skills you will learn and practice in this workbook might help.

SEXUAL SATISFACTION

Sexual satisfaction can play a key role in a woman's quality of life. The aspects of sex that make a woman feel sexually satisfied can include having sex as often as she prefers and, during sex, experiencing sexual pleasure and feeling emotionally connected to her partner. Satisfaction is not simply a lack of dysfunction. In fact, a woman who experiences sexual difficulties might still feel sexually satisfied, which suggests that the factors that contribute to sexual satisfaction are different from those that contribute to sexual function. Satisfaction is related more to quality than frequency of sex. So, even if you experience problems with sexual desire, arousal, or orgasm, you could still feel sexually satisfied if sexual activity brings you a rewarding outcome, such as a deeper level of emotional connection with your partner during, or even days after, sex.

It is important to think about what makes sex satisfying for you. Does it hinge on a certain experience, like orgasm? What would it be like to let go of some of the traditional markers of sexual satisfaction (e.g., orgasm) and explore what else could make sex satisfying for you? The mindfulness practices that you will learn about in this workbook might help you to uncover what makes sex satisfying to you.

HOW COMMON ARE SEXUAL DIFFICULTIES?

Any aspect of sexual response can become a problem—either on its own, or together with problems in other areas of sexual response. Over the past decade, a number of large surveys of representative samples of women across a diversity of ages, cultures, socioeconomic backgrounds, and other indicators of identity and social situation have explored how common various sexual difficulties are and what factors make women more likely to have a sexual problem.

Reduced or absent sexual desire is consistently the most common sexual difficulty that women report, with one-third of women saying that this has been an issue for them for at least three months over the past year. This rate increases with age. The increasing rates of sexual problems as people age have been attributed to changes in physiological response in the body, overall health declines, problems in the relationship in general, or a partner's sexual dysfunction; however, it also seems that these increasing difficulties level off when people are aged fifty-five to sixty-four. Difficulties with orgasm are also fairly common, with about one in five women reporting this difficulty over the past year. Slightly fewer women experience pain with sexual activity. When this occurs chronically with no other obvious explanation (like a yeast infection or a skin condition), it is diagnosed as Provoked Vestibulodynia, as discussed earlier in this chapter.

Up to 8 percent of women report being anxious about sex. Some express a fear of sexual activity because of a concern that sex might hurt; others might have had unwanted sexual encounters in the past that gave rise to feelings that sex is frightening. As a result, these women avoid not only intercourse but also any activity that could lead to sexual activity, such as foreplay, kissing, holding hands, or undressing in front of a partner.

In a large US survey led by the research scientist Debra Herbenick in 2019, a total of 24 percent of women (compared with 10 percent of men) reported that they had felt scared during sex at any time in their life. Examples of what made sex scary included being forced into sex, or being held down, being threatened, or experiencing pain during sex.

IS EVERY WOMAN WHO HAS SEXUAL DIFFICULTIES BOTHERED BY THEM?

Some women have sexual difficulties only in one aspect of their sexual response, whereas others experience sexual difficulties in many domains. Not all women who have sexual difficulties are distressed by them, though. Only one in three women who have difficulty with sexual desire (or 10 percent of the adult population) report feeling distressed by their low desire.

This means that two-thirds of women with low desire might have an explanation for their low desire that makes sense to them and means they do not feel distressed about their low desire. For example, a woman who is dealing with a significant life stressor might feel her reduced desire is perfectly natural given her current situation. Some women might not feel distress because their sexual difficulty does not interfere with their relationship. Others might have adapted to the sexual difficulty so that it does not create a significant problem for them.

We're all different, of course, and so some women are more likely than others to be distressed or bothered by their sexual difficulty. Researchers have sought to identify these women and the factors that play a role in their responses to their difficulty. It turns out that expectations play a significant role in how women respond to sexual difficulties. Women who feel they should have a much higher level of sexual desire or response than they actually experience are more likely to be bothered by their "inadequate" sexual desire. This speaks squarely to the need for women to have realistic expectations about sexual response (and sexual activity), since an unmet expectation can be a source of distress. Women who struggle with depression or poor self-image are also more likely to be bothered by a sexual difficulty. It is possible that feelings of helplessness (such as feeling that they cannot improve their situation) contribute to the feeling that their sexual concerns are unsolvable, which in turn leads to more distress. We also know that low mood in general and the apathy that often characterizes depression can lead to more distress in women with a sexual difficulty.

Women who report that they have decreased physical sensations or reduced pleasure during sex are also more likely to be distressed by their sexuality. This makes sense, because for many women, the desire for sex is related to feeling good during sex, and if pleasure is reduced, the motivation for sex is also reduced, which can be distressing to some women. For many (perhaps even most) women in long-term relationships, sexual desire emerges after they feel arousal in a sexual encounter.

In other words, although a woman might not be motivated to have sex at the outset, if she is sexually stimulated and arousal sets in and she continues to focus on that arousal and it feels good, desire might emerge. If arousal is impaired (say, for a medical reason or because of menopausal symptoms), however, or the physical sexual response does not feel good, she might not experience responsive sexual desire. In such situations, it makes sense that a woman would feel distressed by her lack of both arousal and desire.

Women who can identify a reason, or reasons, for their sexual concern are less likely to experience distress. For example, a woman who speculates that her low desire might stem from a lack of adequate sex education as a child or a negative sexual experience as a teenager or a chronic medical health issue or ongoing daily stress has identifiable reasons for her low sexual motivation. She is therefore less likely to be distressed than a woman who cannot identify any "reasons" for her low desire. Chapter 2 provides a framework for considering some events in your own personal life and relationship that might have contributed to a sexual difficulty.

CAN MINDFULNESS HELP ALL SEXUAL DIFFICULTIES?

Much of our research has been focused on mindfulness as a tool to improve problems with sexual desire. The skills I introduce in this workbook will be helpful across the range of all aspects of sexual response, function, and mood, not just sexual desire. I will go into more detail in later chapters to illustrate this point.

STRUGGLES AND STRATEGIES

Encountering challenges as you embark on a journey of mindfulness is very common and is most definitely not a sign that you are not benefiting from it or that you are not able to learn mindfulness. It is also not a sign that your sexual issues are too severe, longstanding, unusual, or complex to be improved through mindfulness. Encountering challenges is a sign that you are human and live in a world full of complexity and challenges. Show compassion to yourself when (not if) you face struggles.

Below are eight common challenges many people experience when they embark on a mindfulness program. Read through each one and ask yourself if you can relate to them as you begin to undertake the exercises in this workbook. You can add other strategies to this list if any come to mind as you work through the exercises.

THE STRUGGLE: RELUCTANCE

You are wary of putting in the effort required for this kind of program. You might not sense any feelings of joy or hope that the future will be different after you have worked through these exercises.

Strategies

· Remind yourself that there is solid scientific evidence that these skills work! Research has demonstrated that regular mindfulness practice can significantly boost many aspects of sexual desire, satisfaction, and pleasure, and reduce feelings of stress, anxiety, and depression.

· Be gentle and compassionate to yourself about your reluctance. It is fine and even common to be skeptical. Try to bring an openhearted friendliness to those feelings.

· Just do the best you can and gently notice judgments that arise about your degree of effort, perhaps saying to yourself, "A-ha! I notice that I am judging myself for not trying more." Adjust your expectations around effort.

THE STRUGGLE: FORGETFULNESS

You find yourself forgetting what to do while practicing mindfulness. Maybe you repeatedly get lost in the content of your thoughts rather than observing the flow of your thinking. Maybe you forget to come back to what you were focusing on in your practice and instead let your mind drift where it wants to go.

Strategy

· Do it anyway! The more you practice mindfulness, the less likely you will be to experience periods of being "lost in thoughts." Thoughts will always be there, and with practice you will be able to notice them without getting pulled into the endless rabbit hole of one thought leading to another.

THE STRUGGLE: FEELING TIRED

You are feeling too mentally exhausted to do any mindfulness practice. Within a few minutes of beginning a meditation, you fall asleep.

Strategies

· Reframe your mental tiredness as a reminder to practice because you know that mindfulness is an effective way of cultivating mental wellness. Reframing the fatigue as a reminder rather than a struggle for practice sounds difficult, but it works!

· Keep in mind that our practice is about "falling awake," not "falling asleep." Thus, if ways of practicing that support an alertness during practice, such as keeping your eyes open, do not prove helpful, you might wish to defer your practice until you are more rested.

THE STRUGGLE: FEELING TOO STRESSED OR ANXIOUS

Some people experience an increase in stressful feelings or even anxiety when they meditate. This does not mean that you are doing something wrong or that mindfulness is not working for you. In fact, it could be a sign that you are doing everything just right by carefully paying attention to your physical sensations. For some people, thinking about carving out thirty minutes in their day to practice can also cause stress as it becomes "yet another thing on my to-do list!"

Strategies

· See if you can bring mindful awareness to the anxious feelings by noticing the bare sensations that make up anxiety. Sometimes when we label something (as anxious, painful, disliked), the label can make the feelings seem a lot worse. Rather than labeling, use your mindfulness skills to move even closer to the individual sensations that make up the anxiety (such as rapid heart rate, warmth, pressure) and breathe through them.

· Mindfulness practice is not meant to be stressful. If you put it on your to-do list, take something else off. Also, remind yourself that mindfulness is one of the best ways to manage stress in your life, so the short-term investment in practice could have long-term benefits for you.

THE STRUGGLE: STRIVING TOO HARD TO "MEDITATE PROPERLY"

Many people are perfectionists, but this can backfire. If you get distracted during a mindfulness practice, you might tell yourself that "you're doing everything wrong" and "you just need to try harder." This striving can make your mindful practice even more challenging. Plus, perfectionism is an illusion.

Strategies

· Putting in the right effort is key to effective mindfulness practice. Too much effort can contribute to a sense of restlessness when you practice, and too little can contribute to sleepiness. Imagine holding a delicate flower in your hand. If you hold it too loosely, it might fall to the ground, but if you grasp it too tightly, the petals might fall out. In mindfulness practice, you want to bring the right amount of gentle attention to your moment-to-moment experiences with just enough effort to allow your attention to rest on sensations, but not so much effort that your attention lands too heavily and gets stuck on a particular sensation.

· Let go of perfectionism. Remind yourself that the goal of these practices is to bring a gentle, kind attention to present-moment experience. You are not striving for the "perfect" experience or the "right set of sensations." Being aware of your inner critic allows you to realize how much we all live inside our heads, immersed in memories of the past or in ideas about an imagined future.

THE STRUGGLE: "GIVING IN" TO THE TEMPTATION TO FOLLOW DISTRACTIONS

Getting distracted by other thoughts or sounds while practicing mindfulness is common and does not mean you're "doing it wrong." When this happens, guide your attention back to the present moment. Sometimes you don't realize this until many minutes have passed, though. You might not realize you've been distracted until your meditation practice ends.

Strategies

· Forgive yourself. It's tough to break the habit of living in the past or the future. Many people spend most of their time in planning mode, or in past memories mode, so refocusing on the here-and-now takes much effort and time. However, it can be done with consistent practice. Being compassionate with yourself will allow you to move on and follow this practice, even if you have not been consistent in your mindfulness practice. Noticing judgmental thoughts that you are a "failure" or "bad" or inadequate in some way does not mean that you are any of these things.

· Even if you get distracted for the last fifteen minutes of a mindfulness practice, set an intention in your next practice to reduce this to ten minutes of distraction, and then five minutes, and eventually, you'll be able to notice immediately when your mind "takes off" and to bring it back.

THE STRUGGLE: BEING PHYSICALLY TOO TIRED

For many people, mindfulness practice takes a lot of physical effort (as well as mental and emotional effort). Sitting upright in a chair for thirty minutes without back or neck support can be very challenging. Also, some standing mindful stretching exercises can elicit muscle fatigue.

Strategies

· Remember that cultivating mindfulness can provide you with physical energy, so try to practice even when you're feeling physically tired.

· It might be tempting to practice the mindfulness skills only before bedtime to help you fall asleep. Although relaxation skills can be very useful for helping overcome sleep difficulties, in this case you want to fall awake. Also, try to not do any of the mindfulness practices in the bedroom, as good sleep hygiene practices mean reserving the bedroom for sexual activity and sleep.

· If any of the instructions elicit too much physical discomfort, simply modify them! You can do the mindful stretching while sitting down. And for the sitting practices, you can rest your back and neck against the back of a high-back chair or sofa to provide the needed support. If you deal with chronic pain, make any adjustments you need at the start of and throughout the practice.

THE STRUGGLE: NOT SEEING IMMEDIATE BENEFITS

When you invest time in a new program, it is natural to expect to see improvements. If you don't see any improvement right away, you might feel impatient or frustrated. This is fairly common when people begin a mindfulness program.

Strategies

· Learning any new skill takes time. For many of you, mindfulness skills will be an entirely new skill set to develop. The goal of these exercises is to develop skills to be present with moment-to-moment experience, which includes noticing the temptation to look for improvements right away.

- We often tell participants in our groups, "If you are unhappy with point A and really want to get to point B, the way you will get there is by remaining at point A." (Yes, you read that correctly.)

- Be patient, and rather than focusing on progress, focus on practice.

TIME TO PRACTICE

Over the next week, I invite you to practice mindful eating every day as your informal practice. Set aside ten minutes a day to do this. You can use any food item you like. Use a log to track your practice and make any observations about it.

Choose a ten-minute period for your mindful eating practice. Decide beforehand to not answer the phone, respond to texts, and so on during this time. Begin by noticing the sensations of being seated in a chair and your general level of energy, stress, and sense of time for your practice. Congratulate yourself for taking these ten minutes to practice the mindfulness skill of attention regulation.

Then bring a gentle, curious attention to the visual qualities of the food item, noticing its color and texture, and how the light plays on the surface. Pick up the food item (with your fingers or cutlery) and notice its weight, or texture, or both. Lift the item to your nose and notice any scent. Also carefully notice thoughts when they occur, and then bring your attention back to the sensations associated with the food item.

Notice when you make a decision to place the food in your mouth and bring attention to how that decision is translated into movement. Also bring attention to any ways that your body prepares to receive the food. Bring attention to placing the food in your mouth, noticing sensations of texture, taste, and temperature. Bring a friendly interest to the sensations associated with chewing and swallowing. Continue to notice and acknowledge any thoughts, without doing anything to deliberately alter them.

Pay attention to as much detail as possible of the physical sensations and bring a kind curiosity to the experience (e.g., "Are there any other physical sensations occurring that I have not noticed yet?"). Perhaps ask yourself, "Do I experience some of the sensations as pleasant? Unpleasant? Neutral?"

At the end of the ten-minute practice, thank yourself for taking the time to practice mindfulness. Perhaps form the intention to bring a friendly interest to noticing sensations at other times of the day as well.

2

The Body Scan Foundation for Mind-Body Sex

FORMAL EXERCISE 2:
THE BODY SCAN PRACTICE

The Body Scan practice is used in many mindfulness-based programs. It involves paying attention to one part of the body in great detail, noticing all of the individual bare sensations in that region, and then moving on systematically to all other parts of the body.

It is not an exercise to relax the body. And it is not the same as progressive muscle relaxation, which involves first tensing and then relaxing the major muscle groups in the body in turn to induce greater relaxation. Although many people experience the Body Scan as relaxing, the goal is to bring the same moment-by-moment attention to the different parts of the body as you did when you were mindfully eating the raisin or other piece of food.

Sometimes bringing awareness to a part of the body can make you "think" about that area. This is not the goal either. When you are focusing on the sensations of the foot, you are not *thinking* about the foot, having memories of the foot engaged in activities, or trying to create sensations in the foot by moving it in any way. Rather, you are simply bringing your awareness to any sensations that are there in the region of the foot.

Sometimes this entails noticing *no sensations* too. As strange as that sounds, you can notice the absence of sensations, and you will get a lot of practice doing that during the Body Scan. During sexual or other activities, the body sometimes simply does not produce sensations that you notice. If you can accept that fact, you are less likely to become alarmed or distressed if it happens during sexual activity.

I recommend taking a seated position for this Body Scan, although some people prefer to do it lying down. If you have discomfort or chronic pain, feel free to lie on a bed or couch or yoga mat. If not, try to sit in a high-back chair that has lower back support. The room should not be too hot or too cold. For extended mindfulness practices, some people like to cover themselves with a blanket. Most important of all, make sure your phone and any other device that produces vibrations is turned off. If you plan to listen to the audio recording of the Body Scan instead of reading the instructions below, simply turn off the notifications for incoming calls or messages on your electronic device.

In this practice I will invite you to close your eyes, but this exercise is about falling awake, not falling asleep, so if you feel a tendency to doze off, either keep your eyes open or open them periodically throughout the meditation.

WHAT YOU WILL NEED

- A chair (ideally high-back) or yoga mat
- A quiet space (remember that no space will be totally silent, and that is okay!)
- Your journal

This practice will take about twenty-five minutes.

STEP-BY-STEP GUIDE TO THE BODY SCAN

- To begin, settle into a comfortable sitting position, with your feet flat on the floor and legs uncrossed. If you're lying down, keep your legs parallel.

- Allow your back to adopt an erect, dignified posture, with your spine, neck, and head in alignment and your hands resting on your thighs or in your lap.

- Allow your eyes to close if this feels comfortable. If not, you can leave them open or open them at any point during this practice with a soft, unfocused downward gaze.

- Set an intention for this practice. Perhaps it is to allow yourself to fully notice sensations in your body. Perhaps it is to be open to whatever comes up during the practice. Perhaps your intention is to be kind to yourself when your attention gets pulled away. You might also set more than one intention for this practice.

- Do your best to stay alert and mentally focused throughout the practice. Your only goal is to become aware of whatever sensations are present in different parts of your body in each passing moment and to bring an accepting attitude toward whatever arises in your field of awareness, looking at it clearly and seeing it as it is.

- Whether your experience is positive, negative, or neutral, this is your present reality and you are going to simply notice it. Allow yourself to be exactly as you are.

- As you progress through the different parts of the body, do not try to change what you are experiencing. You are not trying to become more relaxed or less tense. Tension, restlessness, and doubt can all be experiences that you observe, just as you are observing sensations in your body.

· Throughout this Body Scan it is likely that there will be things that capture your attention, such as a physical sensation in another area of your body, a sound, or a thought that becomes predominant. Allow this to be the new focus for your attention for a moment and bring the same level of mindful awareness to it as you brought to your body earlier in your practice, continuing to observe it until it is no longer predominant. Then bring your attention back to your breath and to the region of your body you are focusing on.

· Remember that there are no "correct" sensations that you should experience. Give yourself permission to notice what is occurring moment to moment without needing to change it in any way.

· First, bring your attention to the sensations of contact between your body and the chair and the floor—all those places where your body is supported as you sit here. Notice any sensations of touch or pressure.

· Next, slowly bring your attention to the sensations of breathing. You should not manipulate your breath in any way, such as trying to make it slower or deeper, but simply experience the sensations of breathing as the air moves in and out of your body. Direct attention to your abdomen and feel the sensations in that region as the breath comes into your body and your abdomen gently expands, and as the breath moves out of the body and your belly deflates.

· Allow your attention to rest on sensations of breathing moment to moment. Follow with your mind's eye the rhythmic movements of your belly with each breath. Notice the rising of your belly on the in-breath and the falling of your belly on the out-breath.

· Over the next few breaths, gather your attention and move it down the left side of your body, down the left leg, all the way to the toes of your left foot. Allow your attention to rest on whatever sensations are in this region of the toes right now. There might be sensations of contact, tingling, moisture, itching, or warmth or coolness.

- The specific sensations are not important in themselves. Just bring your attention to your toes as they are. If you find that no sensations are present in this region, just experience "not feeling." What is it like to not feel sensations? Feel the big toe as it is, and the little toe, and then the toes in between.

- When you are ready, perhaps on an out-breath, release your attention from your toes and move it to the bottom of your left foot—the ball of your foot, the heel, and the arch.

- Notice places of contact with your shoes or socks or the floor and sensations of touch or pressure. Bring a gentle, curious attention to the entire sole of your left foot. Observe it just as it is.

- When you are ready, release your attention from the bottom of your left foot and move it up to the top of your left foot and your ankle. Become aware of any sensations on the surface of your skin and deep inside, all the way down to the bones. Become aware of the top of your left foot and ankle and whatever sensations or lack of sensations are there. You are not "thinking" about this region but just noticing sensations there.

- You may find yourself engaged in or identifying with the content of a thought. When this happens, just gently acknowledge that this has happened and guide your attention back to the region you were focusing on.

- When you are ready, release your attention from the top of your left foot and ankle and move it to your left lower leg and knee. With patience and kindness, see if you can notice sensations in your shin in the front and your calf muscles in the back.

- Notice your kneecap, the knee joint, the back and sides of your knee. Notice not only the surface but also deep down to your bones.

- Experience the entire lower leg. Don't try to make it be any different from what it is. Just accept the sensations that you observe. You might even say, "Ah, here you are..."

- When you are ready, release your attention from your left lower leg and knee and move it up to the left upper leg, the thigh, and finally the groin. See if you can detect sensations of contact with the chair and your left hand or arm resting on your thigh. Notice sensations in the muscles and bones of your left thigh.

- When you are ready, release your attention from your left thigh and move it up to your left hip and then across your body to your right hip, and then all the way down your right leg to the toes of your right foot.

- When you reach your toes, notice whatever sensations are present in your big toe and little toe and the toes in between.

- Breathe.

- Just register the sensations in this region. Try not to judge them or worry about what your toes should feel like. Allow them to be exactly as they are.

- When you are ready, release your attention from your toes and move it to the bottom of your right foot, including the ball of your foot, the heel, and the arch. Expand your attention to include the top of your right foot and ankle. Try to feel the entire right foot and ankle.

- When you are ready, release your attention from your right foot and ankle and move it up to your lower right leg and knee. Notice your shin in the front and your calf muscles in the back, then the kneecap, the knee joint, and the back and sides of your knee. Perhaps notice sensations on your skin, or notice a lack of sensations in certain areas or at certain times throughout your mindfulness.

· When you are ready, release attention from your lower right leg and knee and move it up to your upper right leg, your thigh, and all the way up to your groin. Observe sensations of contact with the chair and your right hand or arm resting on your thigh. Notice sensations in the muscles and bones of your right thigh. Move your attention deep into your groin.

· When you are ready, release your attention from your right thigh and groin and move it up to your right hip and left hip and the entire area of the pelvis, from one hip to the other. Spend a moment noticing sensations in your pelvis and lower abdomen and your buttocks.

· Notice sensations of contact with the chair and your thighs. Become aware of the region of your genitals and any sensations that are there in this moment. Warmth? Dryness? Wetness? Pulsing? Numbness?

· Try to move your attention even closer to the different parts of your genitals: the labia majora (outer lips), labia minora (inner lips), mons, clitoris, and vagina. Can you sense the area of tissue between the vagina and anus, called the perineum? Don't "think" about that region, but just sense it. As it is.

· Notice if the sensations are accompanied by a pleasant, unpleasant, or neutral feeling. Are there any thoughts in your mind? If so, and as best as you can, simply allow even judgmental or critical thoughts to be there without reacting to them or judging yourself for having them.

· Bring the same gentle acceptance to your thought sensations that you have been bringing to your physical sensations.

· When you are ready, release your attention from your pelvis and move it to your lower back. Notice any sensations of contact with the chair and any subtle movements in your lower back associated with breathing. Notice any sensations of tightness or tension.

· This is an area in which we often store tension. Just allow yourself to feel whatever sensations are there. If you find yourself having thoughts about pain or discomfort, acknowledge that those thoughts are there and let them be. Then try to move back to the bare sensations themselves. Just experience sensations in your lower back as they arise, linger, and move on.

· When you are ready, move attention from your lower back to your abdomen. See if you can just feel the rising and falling of your belly as you breathe. Allow your awareness to expand from the belly up to your chest. Feel the movements of the diaphragm, that umbrella-like muscle that separates the abdomen from the chest, heart, and lungs. Experience the chest as it expands and contracts on the out-breath.

· Notice any sensations associated with the rhythmic beating of your heart within your chest. Pause and observe any feelings arising from your chest and belly—the entirety of the front of your body.

· When you are ready, release your attention from the front of your body and move it around to your upper back and shoulders. Just feel the sensations in this region: the rib cage expanding on the in-breath and contracting on the out-breath. Notice any sensations comprising a feeling of tension or relaxation, of tightness or ease in your upper back and shoulders, and notice any associated feelings of liking or disliking these sensations, either wishing they would stay or wishing they would go away. Notice any thoughts and bring a gentle acceptance to those that may be arising, lingering, and then moving on.

- When you are ready, release your attention from your upper back and shoulders and move it down your left arm to the finger-tips of your left hand. Become aware of the sensations in the tips of your fingers and thumb, and perhaps also any dampness, warmth, or pulsations from the blood flow.

- Expand your awareness to include your entire left hand: the back of your hand, the palm, and the wrist. What sensations do you notice there?

- When you are ready, release your attention from your left hand and wrist and move it up to your left forearm and elbow and your upper arm—the entire left arm all the way up to the arm-pit. Bring a gentle and kind attention to all sensations in your left arm. Notice sensations that are there as well as an absence of sensations.

- When you are ready, release your attention from your left arm and move it across your body and down your right arm to the fingertips of your right hand. Become aware of the sensations in the tips of your fingers and thumb. Expand your awareness to include your entire right hand, the back of the hand and palm of the hand, and the right wrist. Can you sense feelings in this area?

- When you are ready, release your attention from your right hand and wrist and move it up to your right forearm and elbow and your upper arm—the entire right arm all the way up to the arm-pit. Bring a gentle and kind attention to all sensations in your right arm.

- Acknowledge if your mind has drifted elsewhere and gently guide it back. You may have to do this many times, and that is okay.

- When you are ready, release your attention from your right arm and move it up to your neck, including the back of your neck and your throat. Experience sensations in your swallowing and breathing.

- When you are ready, release your attention from your neck and move it up to your lower face. Bring your attention to your jaw and chin, your lips and mouth, then to your teeth and gums, tongue, the roof of your mouth, the back of your mouth, and your throat.

- Expand your awareness up the face to include your upper lip, nose, cheeks, eyes, and eyelids, as well as your eyebrows and the space between the eyebrows, your temples, and your forehead. Allow your attention to rest on your entire face, just as it is here and now. It does not need to be any different.

- When you are ready, release your attention from your face and move it up to the top of your head and the back and sides of the head, including your ears—the entire cranium and the space inside your head as well.

- When you are ready, expand the field of your awareness to include your entire body, from the top of your head to the soles of your feet. Pay careful attention to the many individual sensations that arise and pass away within this larger field of awareness, wherever they are located in your body.

- Allow your attention to move fluidly from sensation to sensation, wherever they arise, momentarily focusing on each one as it rises and then fades, and, without straining, observe each sensation as clearly as possible.

- As you come to the end of this practice, perhaps form the intention to bring this moment-to-moment noticing of sensations to the rest of the day.

- You may wish to wiggle your toes and fingers, noticing sensations of movement. You may wish to congratulate yourself on having taken the time and applying the energy to nourish yourself in this way and to remember that this state of awareness is accessible to you by simply attending to sensations, such as those of the in-breath and the out-breath, in any moment, no matter what is happening, at any time of the day.

- Whenever you're ready, allow your eyes to open if they were closed. If your eyes remained open, you can now lift your gaze straight in front of you. Shift your focus from physical sensations to a deeper consideration of your experiences as you carry out the Inquiry.

- If you were lying down during the Body Scan, now is a good time to sit upright.

- Finally, take a few deep breaths before you move on to the Inquiry.

THE INQUIRY

Now spend the next ten to fifteen minutes reading and answering the three Inquiry questions—possibly more if there is a lot to notice! You can say your answers aloud, write them down in your journal, or simply reflect on them. Whichever option you choose, though, take the time to consider each question in *detail*.

QUESTION 1. What did you notice during the Body Scan?

Consider what sensations arose during this practice. Focus on the "bare sensations" you noticed rather than interpreting the sensations or making inferences about how this practice might help your sexuality. What other sensations were you aware of? Can you describe those feelings in detail? How long did each sensation last? How long did the sensation following each one last? What else came up for you as you observed the different parts of your body? Were there areas of your body where you did not notice any sensations? What was that like? Did you sense an urge to move your body in a particular way? Did you notice restlessness, and if so, how did you experience that in the moment? How did you handle distractions?

QUESTION 2. How was paying attention to your body, in the way you just did, different from how you normally observe sensations in your body?

How was noticing the sensations in your feet, arms, back, neck, abdomen, and head different from how you normally observe feelings in those body parts? Try to be as detailed as possible about how this experience was similar to or different from how you typically notice sensations in your body. In what ways was it different? In what ways was it similar? Again, take at least five minutes to consider each of these questions.

QUESTION 3. How was this exercise relevant to your sexuality?

How was observing your body, part by part and with nonjudgmental awareness, relevant to your sexual desire or sexual arousal? How was the attention you harnessed during this exercise important for understanding your sexual response? What learnings can you take from this Body Scan to apply to your sexual health? How can this practice of mindfully observing your bodily sensations be used to improve aspects of your sexual life? Remember that there is no single correct answer. Any observation you make is useful and important. Again, take at least five minutes to consider each of these questions.

END OF THE BODY SCAN PRACTICE
You have just completed the formal Body Scan and Inquiry. Now might be a good time to stand and stretch before continuing. Congratulate yourself for completing what might be your longest mindfulness practice to date.

The Body Scan is a staple of our mindful sex program, and we have introduced it to many hundreds of women over the past several years. Each time I ask the Inquiry questions I am awed by the curiosity, wonder, and discovery that the women describe as they notice their bodies. In response to question 1 (What did you notice during this practice?), our past mindful sex group participants have shared the following:

- I have never focused on sensations in my toes before. That was a first for me!

- I noticed that tension in my neck is actually made up of many different sensations—some of which are uncomfortable and some of which are neutral.

- I noticed myself wanting to stretch or relax or tense certain parts of my body where I couldn't feel any sensations.

Overall, the Body Scan practice might lead you to feel sensations that are new, unfamiliar, strange, welcome, or surprising. Many people discover that each sensation is not static or singular. Sensations are made up of a multitude of smaller individual sensations that vary in their frequency and intensity.

When I have asked our group participants how paying attention to their body in this way is different from how they normally notice their body (question 2 of the Inquiry), some say that they can sense their breathing in many different parts of the body or that a large range of different sensations accompanies the breathing. It is not just air moving! They notice pressure, a lightness, a relaxation, points of tension, vibrations, and even a temperature associated with those sensations of the breath.

Others say that a part of their body where they usually feel pain could be "just observed" in the Body Scan, without them being pulled into the discomfort of and emotions associated with pain. They could just *be* with those sensations of pain without reacting to them. Some comment that paying attention to each part of their body helped them appreciate the many parts of their body that they otherwise ignore and that spending equal time with each body part helped them feel that they were nourishing their entire body, not just the parts that always call for their attention. Still other women state that they never pay attention to their physical sensations unless there is a problem and that taking the time to notice their body when it is "neutral" was refreshing for them.

In sum, few of us pay much attention to our bodies unless there is pain or discomfort, and even then, our attention is focused only on the source of the pain. Paying attention to all parts of the body, with equal attention and openness, as you did in the Body Scan, offers a very different way of noticing the body from what we do in our day-to-day lives.

I have listened to hundreds of women who have shared their observations of noticing the body sensations after a Body Scan, and I am repeatedly struck by the diversity and depth of their observations. It reminds me that each time we practice mindfulness, it is a brand new practice, even if we have done that particular practice dozens of times before. Mindfulness experts refer to this as "beginner's mind"—or the willingness to see everything as if it were the first time. So many contextual and environmental factors can affect what we observe in this particular situation—how well we slept the night before, if or what we ate, our mood, and the noises in the room can all influence what we observe in a mindfulness practice and how often our minds drift away from the body. Each practice is an opportunity to observe something entirely new—and this is part of the power of mindfulness.

When we asked our group participants how their Body Scan practice might be relevant to their sexuality (question 3 of the Inquiry), they shared a range of responses. Here is a selection of those responses:

- Paying attention to my breathing resulted in my taking slower and deeper breaths, which in turn felt relaxing. I could see myself doing this in stressful encounters such as when I am worried about sex!

- I observed that the more I paid attention to a part of my body, the more intense the sensations became. I wonder if I paid attention to arousal building during sex if this might cause the arousal to increase more.

- When I was guided to pay attention to the different parts of my genitals, I found myself feeling sensations in regions that I had no idea were there, and this was while feeling neutral and not turned on! It makes me wonder whether paying attention to the different parts of my genitals during sex might heighten the pleasure for me.

- I felt as though just paying attention to an area was sufficient to elicit feelings there. I would imagine that simply focusing on my body before sex or during foreplay could create sexual feelings there.

In the same way that the answers to the third Inquiry question after the eating meditation allowed women to connect mindfulness to enhanced sexuality, the answers to this question after the Body Scan can bring to life the power of mindful sex. And keep in mind that we have not yet applied mindfulness directly to sex! In observing the sensations of the Body Scan, however, and contemplating how those observations might be applied to sex, the Body Scan practice followed by these Inquiry questions allows women to observe even more deeply and to see the relevance and benefits of mindfulness to their sexuality.

It also roots women's commitment to practice. The Body Scan serves as an anchor for the women in our mindful sex groups and is a practice that they return to over and over again.

When we reassessed the women a year after completing our program, we discovered that most of them had continued to practice the Body Scan regularly. Remember, though, that in each practice you will be observing your body as if for the first time.

HOW MIGHT THE BODY SCAN IMPROVE ASPECTS OF SEXUAL RESPONSE?

In our research, we have studied some of the mechanisms that account for the positive effects of mindfulness on sexual desire and other aspects of sexual function. One of the ways that mindfulness works is by improving your awareness of internal sensations in the body, a phenomenon known as *interoception*. For example, *cardiovascular interoception* refers to your ability to be aware of your heart rate in any given moment. People with a strong cardiovascular interoceptive ability can estimate their heart rate with a high degree of accuracy.

There are different ways of measuring interoception, including asking people to answer questionnaires about whether they sense various feelings in their bodies, such as tension, changes in breathing, and pain. These questionnaires may be an effective method of estimating a person's overall interoceptive ability.

Another way of measuring interoception is with an objective measure like true heart rate. To do this, we measure a person's actual heart rate with an electrocardiogram or other similar instrument, and then ask them to estimate their heart rate. The similarity between the perceived heart rate and actual heart rate is a measure of interoception. This is likely a better way of estimating a person's interoceptive ability, since it involves objective measurement rather than a person's estimate of how interoceptively aware they are. We know that people overestimate their ability to sense their body sensations and that they are less interoceptively aware than they think they are.

In our research, we have found that women whose interoception increases after they participate in our mindfulness program are likely to see more improvement in their sexual desire than women whose interoception does not increase. The mindfulness practices the women worked through likely produced improvements in their general awareness of their bodies, which then translated into increases in their sexual desire. What is less apparent scientifically is whether the women had more awareness specifically of sexual sensations in the body after mindfulness or of all bodily sensations. Were they actually more sexually interoceptive? This is an area that merits further study, but our research to date suggests strongly that the Body Scan results in more awareness of the body's sensations, which can directly improve women's sexual desire.

Other research shows that people with overall low interoceptive ability are more likely to experience depressive symptoms and anxiety than people with greater interoceptive ability, providing another reason we should learn to improve our interoceptive awareness. Depression, anxiety, substance use, and eating disorders have all been associated with difficulties in interoception, implying either that those who lack an awareness of their internal body states are more likely to experience symptoms of anxiety, depression, and other psychological issues or that these psychological issues lead to lower interoception. Again, this area merits further study.

Either way, though, mindfulness training can improve both interoception and psychological symptoms and reduce the likelihood of future depressive episodes in people who have had a history of major depression. Armed with this information, you might want to keep the Body Scan practice handy so you're ready to get more in tune with your internal sensations at a moment's notice!

THE MIND-BODY CONNECTION AND
ITS RELEVANCE TO SEXUAL AROUSAL

What is the relevance of this research for mindful sex? It is possible that repeated practice of the Body Scan leads to greater attunement to physical sensations and increased interoceptive ability. In turn, this enhanced attention might directly improve sexual desire and other facets of sexual response, including your overall sexual experience. If a greater understanding of mechanisms is important to you, the following information might be especially helpful.

Do you ever experience sexual arousal in your body but not in your mind? Perhaps when you watch something erotic on television your body shows signs of sexual arousal—pulsing in the genitals, vaginal lubrication, maybe an increase in heart rate—but your mind is not sexually aroused. Or perhaps you sometimes feel turned off by the scene you are watching? Scientists call this phenomenon *lack of concordance*. In the context of sexual arousal, concordance refers to the degree of agreement between physical arousal (in the body) and psychological arousal (in the mind). Research has consistently shown that women are far more sexually discordant than men, meaning that the degree of alignment between physical and mental arousal is lower for women than for men.

The research shows that, with few exceptions, men have fairly strong agreement between mental and physical arousal; when a man's body is sexually aroused, chances are his mind is too. And vice versa. So, if a man watches something erotic, his body might respond with sexual arousal and his mind with "I feel turned on." As with anything, of course, there are exceptions to this high level of concordance in men, but for the most part and across many different research studies, this kind of mind-body agreement in sexual arousal is fairly consistent in men, regardless of their sexual orientation and who they are attracted to.

What does this have to do with mindfulness and women's sexuality? It turns out that, after women participate in a mindfulness program, they show greater alignment of mental and physical sexual arousal. There is preliminary evidence that these improvements in concordance might also translate into improved sexual response for women, though more research is still needed on this topic.

For the purpose of the practices in this workbook, we can conclude that adopting a regular mindfulness practice allows for greater awareness of physical arousal in the body, including more awareness of sexual feelings in the body, which likely translates into greater awareness of mental arousal in the mind, which elicits sexual desire. Put more simply, awareness translates into arousal, which then triggers desire. It seems like a rather simple formula, doesn't it?

We will go into this arousal-desire pathway in more detail later in this chapter. But first, try the following exercise. It will help you to understand the different aspects of your life that might have contributed to a sexual difficulty.

EDUCATION ABOUT SEX: THE FOUR P'S

We will now consider four P's that are helpful in understanding different contributors to sexual difficulties: precipitating, predisposing, perpetuating, and protective factors. We will consider each one of these separately.

If you experience a sexual difficulty—low sexual desire, loss of sexual arousal, difficulties with orgasm—you might be able to recall specific triggers that led to it. We refer to triggers that are obvious and that lead directly to the onset of a sexual problem as *precipitating events*.

Here are a few examples of precipitating events and some suggestions for how you might bring your attention to them:

- **A period of significant stress.** Stress levels are increasing for people in general. How often have you said, "Hello, how are you?" to someone and they respond, "I am so stressed"? The ubiquitous never-ending to-do list can be one of the most pressing stressors on people and can wreak more havoc on our brains and our bodies than a single traumatic event. That stress might be caused by the sheer volume of things we have to do, rather than by having things to do that are particularly stressful in and of themselves. What are your stressors? Can you recall how they affected your sexuality and when? Write in your journal about stressors in your life that might have triggered a sexual difficulty or a change in your sex life.

- **An illness.** For some people, a sudden illness—for example, a heart attack, a cancer diagnosis, or the onset of diabetes—might trigger the beginning of a sexual difficulty. Think about your own health and whether an illness might have triggered a sexual difficulty for you—perhaps a short-term health issue that was identified and resolved quickly or a longer-term or chronic illness that affected you for some time, perhaps even to this day—and write about this in your journal.

- **Difficult menopausal symptoms.** The *perimenopausal transition* is the period between premenopause and postmenopause, when the body is preparing for postmenopause. This period may be characterized by irregular and infrequent menstrual cycles, hot flashes, night sweats, difficulty sleeping, mood changes, irritability, and changes in your body such as loss of fertility, bone density loss, and changes in your cholesterol levels. Not surprisingly, any of these can negatively affect your sexuality. In addition, decreases in estrogen levels, which are important for maintaining vaginal wall elasticity and lubrication, mean that sexual activity can be painful. If sex hurts, your desire for sex will naturally decrease. Have you had perimenopausal symptoms? If so, write in your journal about how it might have affected your sexual desire and response.

- **Emotional distancing within a relationship.** For many women, sexual desire might be directed toward their partner (or not!). Some experience a very strong link between their feelings for their partner and whether they feel sexual desire for that person. Although there are lots of exceptions to this, many women say that they only feel sexual desire for a partner when they also admire, appreciate, and are attracted to them. If there is emotional distancing in your relationship—for example, if your partner makes you feel bad about yourself, blames you when things go wrong, discourages you from participating in activities you enjoy or that will help advance your career, or displays extreme emotions (like anger) toward you—you might feel less desire to engage in sex with your partner. If you are currently in a relationship, how would you rate your overall emotional satisfaction with your partner? How is your desire for sex affected when you feel less emotionally satisfied? If you experience sexual difficulties, does this coincide with a reduction or loss of emotional satisfaction in the relationship? Write about this in your journal.

- **Partner sexual dysfunction.** A period in which your partner experiences sexual difficulty (whether it is erectile dysfunction, premature ejaculation, delayed ejaculation, or low desire in a male partner, or problems with desire, arousal, or orgasm in a female partner) can have a negative effect on your desire for sex and trigger your own sexual difficulty. For this reason, if you want to improve your own sexual function, try to include your partner (when safe and appropriate) to explore whether they have their own sexual problems. Can you recall whether your partner had some of their own sexual difficulties around the time you noticed a change in your own sexual response? If so, write about this in your journal.

- **Physical changes.** A woman's body is capable of many incredible things. The impact of hormones on a woman's body can be quite dramatic—think, for example, of the growth of breast tissue during puberty, and further growth with pregnancy, just before menstruation, and with lactation. Aging and the perimenopause can also affect the body. Exercise or a change in eating behaviors can induce physical changes in the body. While changes in a woman's body do not necessarily directly affect her sexuality, changes in her body image can impact her sexual desire and arousal. A woman who is very critical of her body might monitor it closely during sexual activity or hide parts of it from her partner, and this can hinder her ability to become sexually excited. Thus, for some women, physical changes can be the trigger for a sexual problem. What are your feelings about your own body? What words do you use? What role has body image, or changes in your body, played in triggering a sexual problem? Record these feelings in your journal.

- **Medications.** Some medications are known to trigger sexual concerns. For example, antidepressants, statins (medications that treat high cholesterol), blood pressure medications, benzodiazepines (used to manage panic attacks or extreme anxiety), and anticonvulsants (used to manage seizures and some types of chronic pain) can negatively affect sexual response to varying degrees in different people. When you think back to the start of your own sexual issues, had you begun a new medication or changed the dosage of one you were already on? Some people also develop sexual problems when they stop a medication, so consider that as well in your reflections in your journal.

- **Substance use.** There has been a lot of research into whether prescription or recreational drugs such as cannabis, heroin, cocaine, and ecstasy can affect sexual function. The consensus is that these drugs can affect sexual function in different ways for different people. Alcohol can also affect sexual response. For most people, moderate amounts of alcohol impair sexual arousal (and even orgasm), and chronic use of alcohol can trigger the onset of a sexual dysfunction. When you consider the timeline of your own sexual concerns, was it associated with substance use or alcohol? If so, write about that in your journal.

- **Psychological issues.** We know a lot about the effects of depression and anxiety on sexual function thanks to considerable research in this area. A major depressive episode can trigger a sexual desire disorder. A panic attack can negatively affect sexual arousal and orgasm. But anger, irritability, low self-esteem, chronic worries, self-doubt, pessimism, guilt and shame, and a range of many other psychological issues can also be associated with the onset of sexual concerns, even if you have not been diagnosed as having a psychological issue. If you are experiencing sexual problems, can you identify a period when you were struggling with a psychological issue such as these, or another one? Write your reflections in your journal.

- **Unwanted sexual activity or abuse.** Tragically, approximately one in three women has experienced some form of sexual abuse or harassment. The majority of women never report the abuse or name the perpetrator, and many do not reveal details of the abuse to anyone. In cases of repeated sexual abuse, the victim might *dissociate* as a way of coping with the abhorrent acts inflicted upon them in the moment. Some continue to experience dissociation, even in everyday or neutral or safe circumstances, because it is a learned coping mechanism for them. Abuse can also be physical, verbal, nonsexual, or emotional. In your journal, write your reflections about any experience of abuse or neglect you might have endured and how it might be associated with your sexual function.

The list above is only a selection of precipitating events. You might have had other experiences much earlier in your life, perhaps during your childhood or adolescence, that predisposed you to a sexual difficulty later in life. Think about situations, people, or events that might have made you vulnerable to developing a sexual problem. These are called *predisposing factors*, the second of the four P's.

The list below shows some factors that might have contributed to your vulnerability to developing a sexual problem. None of them are within your control or ability to change now, as they likely occurred many years (or decades) ago. However, bringing awareness to them can be an important part of the healing process. From a mindfulness perspective, identifying these factors can help you to bring compassion to yourself and accept who you are. This does not mean "coming to terms with" or "accepting" the things that happened to you, but there is real power in just knowing and acknowledging different notable events in your life, including those that brought you suffering.

There might be factors in this list you that you can immediately identify as having "set the stage" in your own sexual journey; there might be others you had never considered as having affected your sexuality. Consider the wide range of possible predisposing factors at play in your life in the same way as you considered the precipitating events.

- **Lack of comprehensive sexual education.** Did you receive the "birds and the bees" talk from a parent or teacher or someone else you trusted when you were a child? Chances are you didn't, or if you did, it might have been just a fraction of what you really needed to know. For many people, sex education consisted of a fear-fueled discussion of the dangers of sex, including unwanted pregnancy and sexually transmitted infections. Most people aged forty or older will say that they do not recall having any sex education that included conversations about pleasure, consent, and communication. However, in some places, including Canada, where I live and work, sex education has improved over the years. In addition to learning about sexual and reproductive health, students these days might receive inclusive and comprehensive education on gender diversity, sexual orientation, sexual identities, and relationship configurations. What was your own sexual education like, and do you think it helped you to feel comfortable and confident in your later sexuality, or did it predispose you to having negative beliefs or feelings about sexuality? Write about this in your journal.

- **Negative family messages about sexuality.** Most parents have never received any training in how to talk to their children about sex, so when a child asks, the parents feel ill equipped to answer. They might convey nonverbally that sex is bad or dirty or wrong, and the child then incorporates that message into their belief system. Some parents have been known to react with horror or disgust if they see their child masturbate. When those children grow up, they report remembering that moment vividly, and they might still feel shame and embarrassment even as mature, educated, and informed adults. Sometimes children pick up negative feelings about sex from observing their parents interact. If they notice a parent evading a kiss, they might get the message that intimacy between partners is never to be displayed. Whether subtle or overt, these kinds of messages between parents can set the stage for potent beliefs about sex that persist throughout a person's life. Write in your journal about your own childhood and what kinds of subtle or overt messages about sex your parents conveyed.

- **Childhood sexual abuse.** In the previous section on precipitating events, I talked about sexual abuse being a trigger for a sexual problem. Experiences of sexual abuse or other forms of unwanted sexual activity as a child can be predisposing factors for sexual difficulty and can instill a feeling of shame or guilt around sex that does not manifest until years later when you become sexually active. Some women discover their history of sexual abuse for the first time as an adult when they are working on another personal or psychological issue. If you feel comfortable, write in your journal about whether you experienced sexual abuse as a child. If so, how do you think it has affected your sexuality?

- **Neglect.** For some people, a period of neglect, whether physical or emotional, in childhood can be experienced as traumatic and affect that person's subsequent relationships as an adult and predispose them to a future sexual problem.

- **Depression.** We have discussed depression and other psychological issues as possible triggers of a sexual concern. If depression is a longstanding struggle for you, it might predispose you to a future sexual concern. Depression can lead you to interpret events through a negative or biased lens or to tend to see things as black or white. If something goes wrong, a depressed person might think, "Nothing in my life ever goes according to plan." Or, if there is a verbal disagreement with someone, a person with depression might be more apt to think, "See? I can't get along with anyone. Even this relationship is not working." Such negative ways of seeing the world might persist over time and predispose a person to interpret sexual events in a far more negative way than a person who does not struggle with depression. Given the well-established link between depression (whether it is experienced early in life or more recently) and sexual desire, it becomes especially important to consider the influence of depression on sexuality in your own life. Did you have experiences of depression early in your life? If so, write about them in your journal.

- **Poor self-image.** Some people struggle from an early age to see themselves—both inside and outside—in a positive light. In extreme cases, this can manifest as a lifetime of low self-esteem, self-doubt, or eating disorders, among other possible outcomes. When this negative view of yourself is so strong that you see everything through the lens of "I am not good enough," it can be very challenging as an adult to acknowledge your self-worth. When others pay you a compliment or point out your positive attributes, you might be quick to contradict them. In the sexual domain, this might mean that you conceal your body from a partner during sexual activity to hide your perceived flaws, or do not believe a compliment from your partner about your sexuality or that they find sex satisfying with you. The pervasiveness of low self-image means that it can persist outside of your conscious awareness and can often go unchallenged. If you have a poor self-image, write in your journal about its possible early origins and how it has affected your sexuality today.

The third P is *perpetuating factors*. These are factors that keep an existing sexual difficulty going. They might not have made you vulnerable to a difficulty in the first place or trigger a difficulty. Instead, they perpetuate the difficulty you already have. Here are some common perpetuating factors:

- **Continuing health problems.** If you are struggling with a new health issue that affects your mobility, elicits pain, interferes with sexual response and desire, or requires treatment with a medication that has known sexual side effects, that issue could perpetuate a sexual concern, even if it did not originally trigger the concern. Can you think of any health issues in your own life that could be perpetuating a sexual problem for you? If so, write about them in your journal.

- **New difficulties in a relationship.** Many women who have a sexual difficulty say that it interferes with their satisfaction with their relationship. For some, the reduction in, or outright cessation of, sexual activity can lead to new conflict in a relationship. Given how significant satisfaction with your relationship is for sexual satisfaction, if your sexual difficulties create conflict in your relationship, they will likely also further worsen your sexual functioning, creating a vicious cycle. Do you have a struggle in your current relationship that contributes to an ongoing sexual concern? If so, write about that in your journal.

- **Stressors.** We often think about stress as a predisposing factor as well as a precipitating factor that triggers the onset of a sexual difficulty. Well, guess what? Stress can also be a perpetuating factor, even if it did not elicit the sexual difficulty in the first place. Whether the stress arises from financial concerns, worries about health, or feeling overwhelmed by work, it causes fundamental changes in our brains and our bodies because of the chronic release of cortisol (the stress hormone). An untreated sexual difficulty can also be a source of great stress to a person's relationship. What stressors do you currently have in your life and how do they affect your sexuality? Reflect on this in your journal.

- **Procrastination.** We all procrastinate. Perhaps procrastination is about getting to that one big project that you have been thinking about for months (or even years). Some of us procrastinate about getting our taxes done. And some women might procrastinate about getting help for their sexual difficulty. They might think to themselves, "I'll get to this when I have more time to devote to it." Or, "Maybe if I wait this out long enough, the issue will resolve itself." Unfortunately, procrastination rarely solves the sexual issue. Instead, it keeps the issue alive and inevitably worsens the situation. Do you procrastinate? In what areas of your life? And does this contribute to continuing sexual concerns for you? If so, write about that in your journal.

There might be many other factors in your life that perpetuate a sexual difficulty. Reflect on the obvious and perhaps more subtle factors that could be keeping a sexual difficulty going and write about them in your journal.

For many of us, it is easier to think about negative factors in our lives that contribute to a sexual difficulty than the positive factors that could potentially help us. However, the fourth P—*protective factors*—offers a buffer against the negative effects of first three P's. Another term for these protective factors is *resilience factors*. Resilience is the ability to rise to your feet after being knocked down. It allows you to find another pathway forward and to grow emotionally from negative or traumatic events.

In the case of a sexual difficulty, resilience might enable you to say, "This is a short-term albeit distressing sexual difficulty, but I have hope for the future and I know I can get past this." Having an early family life that conveyed positive messages about sexuality, that normalized sexual attraction and behavior, and that problem-solved when a sexual issue arose can be a powerful protective factor against negative factors during your early life. Having positive attitudes and accurate beliefs about sexuality, and knowing where to get help if it is needed, can also mitigate other negative forces.

Being comfortable discussing sexuality with a partner is a major predictor of long-term sexual satisfaction and is part of the reason communication is often a staple in all forms of sex therapy. Even if you have not always felt comfortable discussing sex with a partner, you can learn to be more comfortable, and once you start, you will soon realize that the benefits far outweigh the perceived risks of healthy sexual communication. Frank, honest, and pleasure-focused communication with a partner can protect against some of the other negative influences on your sexual response.

Limiting the use of medications or other substances with known sexual side effects can also act as protective factors to promote a healthy sexual response. Think about the protective factors in your life, from childhood until today, that might have mitigated the negative influences of other factors on your own sexuality and write about them in your journal.

STRUGGLES AND STRATEGIES

Here is a list of the struggles you might have with the practices discussed in this chapter and some strategies for dealing with them. If none of the strategies really speak to you, think about what would work for you and write it down.

THE STRUGGLE: FINDING THE BODY SCAN TOO LONG

If you are following along with all of the instructions provided earlier in this chapter, or if you are listening to the audio recording on my website, your Body Scan is likely to last for twenty-five minutes. Some of the participants in our groups who were new to mindfulness found this too long. Some reported getting bored. Others found themselves daydreaming after fifteen minutes. Still others reported feeling aches and pains from holding their position for so long.

Strategies

- The twenty-five-minute Body Scan is a guide, not a rule. It is fine to start out with a twenty-minute or even ten-minute Body Scan and then gradually increase the duration of your practice. When you start to feel bored or distracted by random thoughts, instead of taking it as a sign that the Body Scan is too long, treat it as a great opportunity to observe how easily the mind "takes off." You could become curious about where it goes and how often it goes there over the twenty-five minutes. In other words, when you are feeling bored, frustrated, or impatient, use that feeling as an opportunity to tune in rather than tune out.

THE STRUGGLE: CHALLENGES WITH THE INFORMAL PRACTICE

Over the next week, in addition to the formal practice, I suggest that you bring mindfulness to one activity that you do every day, such as walking. If you are used to walking quickly from point A to point B, or if you usually multitask while walking (e.g., eating or listening to music or talking to someone), this slower, more deliberate and attentive type of daily walk might be uncomfortable for you.

Strategies

- Remember that you only need to engage in this informal mindfulness activity for about ten minutes a day—not all day long! Reminding yourself of this at the outset, perhaps even saying, "It's okay, it's just ten minutes," can be a great way to help keep you focused on this informal skill.

- You are already engaging in this activity anyway, so I am not asking you to add more minutes to your day but rather to do what you are *already doing*—just a bit differently.

THE STRUGGLE: GETTING TRIGGERED WHILE DOING THE FOUR P'S EXERCISE

I am asking you to reflect on the different periods of your life and the events that could have contributed in some way to your current sexual concerns. This could bring up sadness, anger, resentment, regret, or many other emotions about events in your past, whether they were under your control or not. Although there is very little, if anything, you can do to change those events from your past, it is useful to think about them and to consider whether they might be affecting your sexuality today.

Strategy

- Try to look at this exercise as one way of bringing acceptance to those events and memories. This is not the same as "being okay with" what might have happened but rather accepting your emotional reaction to these memories. And once you tune in and become familiar with emotions, even negative ones, they start to lose their hold on you.

TIME TO PRACTICE

There will be two mindfulness practices over the next week: a formal practice and an informal practice. The formal practice is the Body Scan, and the informal one is mindfulness during a regular activity.

This week will be an opportunity to dive into your Body Scan practice. Repeat it every day over the next week. In formal mindfulness-based stress-reduction programs, group participants are encouraged to practice the Body Scan seven days a week for up to forty-five minutes each time. Although this might sound like a lot of time to spend scanning your body, in my opinion the Body Scan is the foundational practice on which many other body-focused mindfulness and sexuality exercises are built. Establishing a solid foundation of practice now is important. Many of us engage in less rewarding or perhaps even meaningless activities (such as scrolling through social media posts) for far longer than the time it takes to do a Body Scan. I will ask you to keep coming back to the Body Scan as you continue to work through this workbook.

Keep a chart with the following headings to track your observations during these daily Body Scans: Date of Body Scan, Time, Physical Sensations Noted During Practice and Associated Reflections, Mental Sensations (Thoughts, Emotions) Noted During Practice and Associated Reflections, Minutes Practiced.

Every day over this next week, I invite you to engage in the informal practice of bringing mindfulness to an event or activity that you normally do in your day. For example, if you walk from the parking lot to the grocery store (or to work, to the gym, to visit someone, etc.), slow down your walk and bring a mindful attention to it. Notice the placement of your feet on the ground. What parts of your foot hit the ground first, second, third, and so on? What sensations arise in those different parts of your feet? How far up your legs do you feel sensations as you walk? Do you notice yourself breathing as you're walking? Try to pay attention to your physical sensations, smells, sounds, and mental sensations (otherwise known as thoughts) as you walk mindfully each day. This exercise is best done if you can choose the same activity every day and bring mindfulness to it consistently for at least ten minutes each time.

3

Moving the Body to Focus the Mind

FORMAL EXERCISE 3:
MINDFUL MOVEMENT PRACTICE

In this exercise you will do some simple stretches while standing. If you have ever taken a class in Hatha yoga, you will see some similarities between that and this Mindful Movement practice: both involve holding your body in particular poses, breath work, and paying attention.

You may wish to do this exercise in your bare feet or socks. We will focus on maintaining a moment-by-moment awareness—one that embodies acceptance and nonjudgment. You will explore your body as it gently moves. You can keep your eyes open or close them—whatever feels comfortable to you.

By incorporating movement into this practice, you can observe your tendency to "strive." This practice is done not with a goal of success but in a spirit of discovery and curiosity about what arises in your body from moment to moment. If you are competing with yourself to hold a pose for as long and as still as possible, you might experience feelings of frustration or competitiveness. As you come close to the boundaries of what feels comfortable in these poses, you have an opportunity to observe your limits and accept them, just as they are.

Let's get to the practice so that you can experience it yourself firsthand!

WHAT YOU WILL NEED

- A chair, ideally high-back, or meditation cushion
- A quiet space where you can stand (remember that no space will be totally silent, and that is okay!)
- Comfortable socks or bare feet
- Your journal

This practice will take about twenty-five minutes.

STEP-BY-STEP GUIDE TO MINDFUL MOVEMENT

- To begin this mindful stretching practice, stand with your feet about hips' width apart, with your knees unlocked so that your legs can bend slightly, and with your feet parallel. Your arms can simply hang by your sides. Keep your head up, with your body upright and erect. You could try to embody a sense of dignity and presence, but don't let your body be stiff. You can let your shoulders drop and relax.

- Before we get started, take the time to remind yourself that the intention of this practice is to become aware, as best as you can, of physical sensations and feelings throughout your body as you engage in a series of gentle stretches.

- You are going to investigate and honor the limitations of your body in every moment. And, as best as you can, let go of the tendency to push yourself beyond your limits, compete with yourself, or think about how others do this practice. If you have any physical problems, give yourself permission to remain still at any point or to move only very slightly, to cultivate awareness of your body whether at rest or in movement.

- Do your best to stay alert and mentally focused throughout the practice.

- As you stand here, focus your attention on the sensations of breathing. Observe the sensations as you breathe in and the sensations as you breathe out. Just notice them.

- When you are ready, on an in-breath, begin to move your arms up slowly, with your fingertips pointing out to the sides. Pause for a moment when your arms are parallel to the floor. Breathe out, and continue on the next in-breath to bring your arms up until your hands meet above your head, all the while feeling the tension in your muscles as they work to lift your arms and then maintain them above your head in the stretch.

- Let your breath move in and out freely at its own pace while you continue to stretch upward, with your fingertips gently pushing toward the sky and your feet firmly grounded on the floor. Feel the stretch in your muscles and joints, all the way from your feet and legs up through your back and shoulders and into your arms, hands, and fingers.

- See if you can maintain the stretch for a time, breathing freely in and out, noticing any changes in the feelings in your body as you continue to breathe and hold the stretch. These feelings may include a sense of increasing tension or discomfort. If so, try to be open to that as well.

- When you are ready, slowly, very slowly, on an out-breath, lower your arms with the wrists bent so that your fingers point upward and your palms are pushing outward until your arms come to rest along the sides of your body. Let your arms just hang from your shoulders.

- From here, gently close your eyes and focus your attention on the movements of your breath and the sensations throughout your body as you stand here. Allow your attention to move fluidly from sensation to sensation, wherever they arise in your body, momentarily focusing on each one, as it rises and fades in prominence—perhaps noticing the contrast between your earlier stretch and the current physical sense of release and perhaps relief associated with standing in a neutral stance with your arms at your sides.

· When you are ready, raise your right arm on an in-breath, allowing it to move past your shoulders and head until your hand and fingers are pointing toward the ceiling. As you stand here, focus on the sensations in your hand. Imagine that there is some fruit floating just slightly above your fingertips, and stretch as if to touch it.

· Move your hand as if picking the fruit, bringing your full awareness to the sensations throughout your body. Notice what happens to the extension of your hand and to your breath if you lift your heels off the floor while stretching up on your tiptoes.

· When you are ready, lower your heels to the floor and slowly lower your right arm until it is resting at your side.

· And then, when you are ready again, on an in-breath, lift your left arm all the way up until your hand and fingertips are pointing toward the ceiling and stretch the side of the body, imagining and reaching for the fruit hanging just above your fingertips again. Lift your heels off the floor to extend the stretch, as you did before. Notice any and all sensations in the body as you move in this way.

· When you are ready, on an out-breath, lower your heels to the floor and slowly lower your left arm until it is resting at the side of your body.

· Just stand there and tune in to the sensations in your body.

- When you feel ready, slowly raise both arms on an in-breath so that they are above your head with the palms facing each other, your arms parallel, and your fingertips pointing to the ceiling.

- And then, when you are ready again, on an out-breath, slowly bend your body over to the left side so that both arms and hands are tilting over your side along with your upper torso, and notice that your right hip is gently jutting out toward the right. Notice what it feels like to form a big curve with your body that extends sideways. Feel the stretch in the right side of your body and the slight compression on the left. Feel the stretch from your feet right up through your torso, arms, hands, and fingers.

- On an in-breath, slowly straighten your body and stand upright, continuing to hold your arms up above your head. On the next out-breath, slowly bend over to your right side and form a curve in that direction.

- Both arms and hands are tilting over, your upper torso is tilting over, and perhaps you notice that your left hip is jutting out slightly to the left. Feel the stretch on the left side of your body and the slight compression on the right side. You can guide your attention to feel the stretch from your feet right up through your torso, your arms, your hands, and your fingers.

- On an in-breath, slowly stand upright with your arms above your head. On the next out-breath, let your hands gently come back down toward the sides of your body and just feel the sensations in your body as you stand in stillness. Perhaps notice changes in temperature in your body, or tingling, or your heart beating, or a sense of relief and release. As best as you can, bring awareness to whatever sensations are emerging in your body right now. Turn toward the sensations as best as you can right here, in this moment.

- Now, on an in-breath, raise your shoulders upward toward your ears as far as they want to go and then move them backward as if attempting to draw your shoulder blades together before you let them drop down completely. Squeeze your shoulders together in front of your body as far as they will go, as if trying to touch them together, while your arms remain passive and dangling.

- Continue to roll through these four positions as smoothly as you can for at least two full rotations. Come to rest in a neutral position.

- Now reverse the direction. Raise your shoulders up to your ears and squeeze them together in front of your body, then drop them down and move them backward and together, in something that might resemble a rowing motion. Continue in this direction for the next few moments.

- And then, in your own time, simply stop and stand in stillness in a neutral posture. You might take note of whether you are liking or disliking any of the sensations arising.

- Now form the intention to softly and mindfully roll your head around, to whatever degree you feel comfortable doing so. Very gently, as if you were drawing a circle with your nose in midair, circle your head in a clockwise direction. Remember to move slowly and to the degree that you feel comfortable. After completing a few circles in this direction, circle your head in a counterclockwise direction. Stop and stand in stillness in a neutral posture. As best as you can, tune in to the sensations in your body. Be aware of the sensations in your body, from one moment to the next.

- Now form the intention to transition to your chair for the sitting portion of this practice. As you move, continue to pay attention. In moving from one location to another, remain as focused and aware as you were for the first part of the practice.

- Allow your eyes to open. Settle into a comfortable sitting position either on a straight-backed chair or on a meditation cushion. As best as you can, have your knees slightly lower than your hips. Make any adjustments that enable you to sit as comfortably as you can with an erect and dignified posture.

- Check to see that your spine, neck, and head are in alignment, and make sure that your feet are flat on the floor if you are sitting on a chair. Let your hands rest on your thighs or in your lap. Allow your eyes to gently close if that feels comfortable, or, if you prefer, choose a spot on the floor about four feet in front of you and focus on it with a soft gaze.

- Settle into the sensations of sitting, just as you find them, right here, right now. Allow your attention to move fluidly from sensation to sensation as each one arises and fades in prominence.

- When you are ready, move your focus of attention from the sensations of your body sitting here to the sensations of breathing. Become aware of each in-breath and each out-breath as they follow one after the other.

- Whenever you notice that your attention has moved to a physical sensation elsewhere in your body, a sound, or a thought—anything that becomes predominant—momentarily let it be the new focus for your attention. When it is no longer predominant, bring your focus of attention back to the sensations of breathing.

- In this practice, although there are a number of places in the body where the breath makes itself known, it is often helpful to follow your breath in only one part of your body.

- Focus your attention now on the patterns of physical sensations at your nostrils, as your breath moves into and out of your body. As you breathe in, feel the sensations at your nostrils as the cooler air is drawn into your body. And then, on the out-breath, feel the sensations of friction or pressure at your nostrils as the warm air leaves your body.

· You do not need to breathe in any particular way or use your breath to get anywhere, such as to a deeper state of relaxation or mental calm. Just let yourself breathe.

· When you are ready, move the focus of your attention down your body to your chest, noticing sensations in this region. Feel the expansion of your chest as you breathe in and the falling away of your chest as you breathe out. Tune in to this gentle rhythm of the rising and falling of your chest as you breathe. Observe the sensations of breathing in this part of your body.

· And then, when you are ready again, move the focus of your attention farther down your body to your abdomen and your belly. Feel the expansion of your belly as it rises on your in-breath and the gentle deflation of your belly on the out-breath. As best you can, keep your attention focused from the moment your breath enters your body on the in-breath to the moment it leaves your body on the out-breath.

· Perhaps notice the slight pauses between one in-breath and the out-breath that follows, and between one out-breath and the in-breath that follows.

· Whenever you notice that you have forgotten about noticing your breath sensations because your attention got lost in the content of a thought, and the next one, and the next one, congratulate yourself for becoming aware of that. It is perfectly okay for this to happen. It's simply what our minds do. It doesn't mean it's a mistake or that you're doing anything wrong.

· Notice what your attention was engaged with and then, with kindness, return your attention to the sensations of breathing in the region you are focusing on. Even if your attention becomes engaged in thoughts a hundred times during this sitting, simply notice this and return your attention a hundred times to the sensations of breathing, without any judgment or blame, and just begin again.

- Use your breath as an anchor to gently reconnect with the here-and-now.

- When you are ready, expand your field of awareness to include your entire body, from the top of your head to the soles of your feet. Pay careful attention to the many individual sensations that arise and fade away within this larger field of awareness, wherever they are located in your body. Allow your attention to move fluidly from sensation to sensation, wherever they are arising in your body, momentarily focusing on each one, as it rises and fades in prominence, and, without straining, observing each one as clearly as possible.

- When we meditate for some time like this, it is not unusual for strong sensations to emerge. You may notice sensations of discomfort, pain, or tensing and find that your attention is repeatedly drawn to these sensations. In this practice, there are a couple of ways of working with such experiences. One way is to form an intention to move or readjust your body. If you choose to do so, as best you can, form an intention to move before actually going ahead and moving. Then, notice the sensations of moving themselves and the sensations following the movement. In this way, your response to strong sensations can be guided by the same principles of choice and awareness that we have been practicing all along.

- The other way of working with strong sensations is to bring your attention right up to—or even into—the region of intensity itself and to meet what you find here with an attitude of openness and curiosity. As best you can, observe with gentle and nonjudgmental attention the detailed pattern of sensations you find here. What precisely do the sensations feel like? Where exactly are they? Do they change over time or move from one part of the body to another? What smaller sensations do you notice that make up the single larger sensation?

· Make the strong sensations the focus of your attention for as long as they are predominant.

· If you notice that your attention has become engaged in the content of a thought, or a story about the sensations, you can always return your attention to the present moment by refocusing on the movements of your breath. Once you have gathered yourself in this way, you can choose whether to stay with your breath as the focus of attention or to return to observing the strong sensations in your body.

· If these sensations fade in intensity, allow your attention to move fluidly from sensation to sensation throughout your body as each one rises and fades in prominence.

· In the final few moments of this sitting, perhaps congratulate yourself for taking the time to practice in this way. Acknowledge that by doing so, you are playing an active role in your own health and wellness. Simply by setting aside the time to be with your experience, meeting it as best you can with a nonjudgmental, interested, and friendly awareness, you will be better able to bring mindfulness to the other activities of your day.

· When you are ready, introduce some movement into your fingers and toes and notice the sensations associated with these movements. Allow your eyes to open and notice the sensations associated with the movements of your eyelids and the visual sensations that follow.

· Finally, take a few deep breaths with eyes open before you move on to the Inquiry.

THE INQUIRY

We will now consider in greater depth what you observed during this mindfulness practice. I will pose three questions, and you can answer out loud if you wish, or you can record your answers in your journal. As in the earlier Inquiries, try to take ten to fifteen minutes to answer the next three questions.

QUESTION 1. What did you notice during this practice?

What sensations came up for you during this practice? As you held your body in certain poses, did you experience any particularly strong sensations? What did you do when you noticed these sensations? Did you ever get lost in thoughts? If so, what did you do then? Could you acknowledge when thoughts were there and then shift your attention back to the bare sensations in your body as you held a stretch? What else came up for you as you held your body in various poses? Did any sensations ever become so intense that you wanted to shift position or stop? If so, what did you do then? Take your time in answering these questions.

QUESTION 2. How was paying attention to your body during this mindful stretching different from how you normally observe sensations in your body?

In this practice you may have felt discomfort. We held some of those poses for a long time! The building tension in your body as you held your hands above your head may have felt uncomfortable, and perhaps even painful. I invited you to just pay attention to those sensations without moving or changing them.

How was noticing discomfort in this way—letting it be rather than wanting it to disappear—different from how you might normally experience discomfort? Try to be as detailed as possible in how this experience was similar to or different from how you typically notice sensations in your body. In what ways was it different? In what ways was it similar?

QUESTION 3. How was this mindful movement exercise relevant to your sexuality?

How was staying with discomfort and choosing to "tune in" rather than "tune out" (or distract yourself) relevant to your sexual desire or sexual arousal? Did you surprise yourself by remaining with that discomfort, and if so, what happened to the intense sensations over time? If you did experience discomfort, and remained with it nonjudgmentally, how do you think this way of being with discomfort might be relevant to your sexuality? Did you learn anything from this mindful movement that could be generalized to your sexual desire? Was there something that you did to remain nonjudgmental while you experienced discomfort that you might try in your own sexual life? If so, what, and how? Take the time to consider these questions. I also invite you to keep contemplating these questions throughout the rest of your day and week.

END OF THE MINDFUL MOVEMENT PRACTICE

You have just completed a formal mindful stretching (or stretch and breath) practice plus guided Inquiry. Now might be a good time to stand and stretch before continuing. As always, congratulate yourself for completing this practice. This is not easy work!

When we lead this mindful stretching practice in our groups, participants often share observations such as the following:

- When I started to feel pain in my arms from holding them up so long, I really wanted to lower them to get some relief. But I decided to follow your instructions and just observe my wish for the discomfort to stop.

- I found that by really tuning in to the discomfort and not labeling it as "pain" I was able to truly feel the sensations there. I noticed warmth, tingling, some vibration, and I could draw an imaginary circle around the area of discomfort in my mind. It wasn't that bad.

Participants also say that paying attention to discomfort in this way is different from how they might usually pay attention to discomfort in their day-to-day lives. Here are some participants' comments:

- When I feel something bad in my body, I immediately look at it, rub it, and try to make it feel better. I have never before attempted to just "observe" it without trying to eliminate it! It is definitely a first for me.

- If my body hurts, it upsets me because I have a belief about myself as being healthy and free of pain. So this practice of just letting the pain be there without getting upset by it was really quite different for me.

The third question of the Inquiry asks group members to contemplate how this practice might be relevant to their sex lives. Here are some comments from participants after they completed the mindful stretching practice:

- Sometimes during sex if I worry that my arousal will turn off and I'll experience pain, I start to really focus on discomfort and I am convinced that this "hyper focus" on the possibility of pain actually brings the pain on! I wonder if just focusing on the sensations themselves, without worrying about whether or not they will lead to pain, might lead to a different experience for me. I will try to guide my attention during sex just to the actual sensations, not my interpretation of them.

- Thinking about my low desire leads me to feel demoralized. I keep engaging in sex, as I believe it is important for my relationship, but while we are having sex, I keep waiting to "feel something" like I used to feel. I never do. And then my attention turns to why am I not feeling like I used to feel, and that leads me to feel even worse. It is a vicious spiral that is really challenging to interrupt. I can see how guiding my attention to what actually is there might be more fruitful than waiting to feel something that is not there. I can give that a try.

HOW MIGHT A MINDFUL MOVEMENT PRACTICE IMPROVE ASPECTS OF SEXUALITY?

It can be very helpful to get to know discomfort intimately, since discomfort is inevitable in our lives. Moreover, our tendency to catastrophize when we feel discomfort might be the real cause of emotional trouble, as well as physical trouble. Catastrophizing about how something feels or how you want something to feel can interrupt your sexual response cycle because it prevents you from attending to the early and emerging signs of arousal, which, if you focus on them, can pave the way for sexual desire. In other words, staying in the present, even when the present moment consists of discomfort, can be an important way to ensure that the brain and body are connected and to allow sexual arousal and desire to unfold.

A major theme in this Mindful Movement practice is acceptance. When you sense discomfort, tension, and tightness, accept them. When you observe the relief and relaxation that occur when releasing a tense hold, accept them. And when you do not observe any sensations at all in particular parts of your body, accept that absence.

Why is acceptance such a powerful force in mindfulness practice? Striving for things to be different creates additional internal tension and distress. When you work hard to make something different, sometimes the effort can leave you further away from your goal. As soon as you accept what is, you leave space for the experience to change.

This is relevant to sexual concerns because they can create a lot of distress. But sometimes, striving to make things different right away can exacerbate your sexual difficulty, as we discussed in the Four P's section in chapter 2. The mindfulness practice you just did introduced you to acceptance of unpleasant, neutral, and pleasant sensations. We will continue to work with this theme over the remaining chapters of this workbook.

You might have experienced another major feeling during your mindful movement practice: impermanence. All sensations and experiences are constantly changing. They are not fixed. They are not permanent. Both positive sensations and negative sensations—such as warmth, comfort, discomfort, tension, and pain—are impermanent. Sometimes, when we do not pay attention to sensations, we feel they will last forever. However, when you apply mindful self-compassion to noticing, you might surprise yourself by experiencing the impermanence of the sensation.

EDUCATION ABOUT SEX: INTRODUCING THE SEXUAL RESPONSE CYCLE

In this section we'll learn about sexual desire in more detail. I have included a model to help you understand sexual desire and how it becomes activated. If you have read *Better Sex through Mindfulness*, you will be familiar with this model, developed by Dr. Rosemary Basson, which is discussed at length there. We will then consider how mindfulness might activate this sexual response cycle to cultivate sexual desire.

As discussed in chapter 1, sexual desire can be difficult to define. If you say, "I have lost my desire," what exactly do you mean by "lost"? For some women it means that they have no interest in sex or that their partners are always the one to initiate sex. For other women, absence of desire might reflect a total lack of any sexual thoughts, fantasies, or sexual daydreams. Other women define loss of desire in still other ways. Research on the nature and expression of women's sexual desire has found that there can be perfectly understandable reasons for this lack of desire. For example, feelings of spontaneous sexual desire decrease with age. They also decrease the longer you are in a relationship. In other words, it is quite common for women to lose some of their spontaneous sexual desire—but the good news is that there is a second type of sexual desire, one that seems to resist these influences of age and length of relationship. It is called responsive desire.

WHY HAVE SEX?

Think about why you might have sex (and I mean sex in the broadest way possible). I suspect that this is not something you have thought about before. Most people don't think about why they act, they just act! What are some of your own reasons for having sex? Write them in your journal. Don't analyze your reasons as you're writing them. Just let them arise.

When we pose that question to large groups of people, we hear a variety of reasons, such as to show love, to feel connected, to celebrate a birthday or other occasion, to make a partner feel desired, to feel "normal" (however they define their sense of "normal"), to achieve an orgasm, or to feel sensual. People provide hundreds of reasons for having sex, but "because I was in the mood / had sexual desire" is often not even on the top 10 list for those in long-term relationships. Not having sexual desire at the start of a sexual encounter is okay. It does not mean anything is wrong. It is common.

But having a reason is important, and that reason should be motivated by wanting to obtain something positive, either for you or your partner or for both of you. Having sex to avoid something negative—like a fight, a conflict, or an unhappy partner—is not a good reason to engage in sex. In fact, having sex to avoid a negative situation can cause resentment in the long term. (Chapter 8 has a longer list of such reasons for having sex that you can read through with your partner.)

Having at least one good reason to engage in sexual activity is often the necessary trigger to move you from the neutral "starting block" toward being receptive. Maybe this receptivity means that you will accept your partner's invitation for sexual activity, or maybe it will cause you to initiate sexual activity. Whether you aim to initiate activity or be receptive to a partner's invitation, I urge you to elicit your reason (or reasons) for having sex. Now ask yourself, "Would I initiate sexual activity with my partner (or myself), or would I be receptive to my partner's sexual advances with this one good reason for sex?"

Next, think about what turns you on. What kinds of touch or stimulation between you and your partner elicit sexual arousal for you? Keep in mind that triggers that elicited arousal in the past might not have the same effect on you today, so try to think about triggers that are effective today. These factors could involve your sense of touch, vision, smell, hearing, or something else, and need not be a certain kind of physical sexual stimulation. For example, some people report getting turned on when their partner does something for them or expresses their desire for them. Some people get turned on by watching an erotic scene in a movie. Still others get turned on by certain smells or sounds. Think about what things trigger your own sexual arousal and list them in your journal.

Knowing what your own sexual triggers are is important because they are necessary for eliciting sexual arousal in both your body and your mind. Sexual arousal is not an automatic reflex. It requires that the right stimuli for you are not only at play but also at the right intensity and for the right duration. Sometimes women do not give themselves permission to explore their own bodies and become familiar with the kinds of triggers that turn them on. That issue is discussed in more detail later in this chapter and in the chapters ahead.

Suppose you have a trigger that makes you sexually aroused. What do you typically do next? Some people might feel their arousal but not act on it. Others might then focus more on their bodies to sense and then enjoy their arousal.

The context around you also matters, and this includes the context between you and your partner, and the larger environment around you while you're having sex. Some things in your environment can facilitate this sexual arousal—for example, having privacy, being free of distractions, and feeling relaxed can dial up the arousal and also allow you to tune in to it in more detail. If you are with a partner, having mutual affection, being attracted to your partner, and feeling conflict-free in the moment can also make you more attuned to your arousal. Other factors in the environment—for example, tension in your relationship, worry that someone might walk in, or distracting sounds or sights in the room—can block your arousal.

Your brain takes the information the trigger provides and your body's response to it and either proceeds with a full sexual response or stops right there. Being focused on the present moment and on your arousal can facilitate a sexual response, whereas being distracted, worried, or hyperattuned to the outcome can act as a barrier to it. The brain is truly the largest sex organ, because it ultimately decides whether your reasons for sex, combined with your sexual arousal triggers, will produce a sexual arousal response or not.

Let's suppose that the outcome is positive. You have a reason for sex. You have an appropriate trigger that elicits your arousal. You can pay attention to the sexual response without getting distracted. In this case, the sexual arousal that is elicited will pave the way for what we call responsive sexual desire. Now you want sex, even if that was not your original reason for participating in sex. Once you are turned on and your body is responding, you might suddenly also sense sexual desire as a reason for sex, in addition to your original reasons. This is responsive sexual desire because it emerged in response to sexual arousal. Sexual arousal triggered sexual desire for you. This is a common, normal form of sexual desire and one that is far more common in longer-term relationships.

If the arousal and desire result in a satisfying sexual encounter for you, you will have a rewarding experience that might increase the likelihood that you will conjure up positive reasons for sex next time! What constitutes a rewarding experience will be different for different people and often even for the same person in different encounters. A toe-curling orgasm might be the rewarding outcome one day, whereas feeling emotionally connected with a partner might be a highly rewarding outcome another day.

Can you think about a sexual encounter where you first had sexual arousal, which then triggered sexual desire? Try to pull that memory up in your mind for a moment. How well does this model fit with your own experiences?

To recap how this cycle works: We need reasons for sex, effective triggers, an environment that supports a sexual response, attention, and brain mechanisms that integrate this information. In this cycle, the outcome is arousal first, followed by responsive desire.

WHEN SEXUAL RESPONSE IS BLOCKED

Can you think of anything that could get in the way of the cycle just described above? Try to identify the different barriers in your own experiences that block this cycle and write them in your journal.

Sometimes a person might not be able to think of any positive reasons for sex because they only want to avoid some anticipated negative outcome (like a fight or ongoing conflict). Engaging in sex to avert an argument, especially if this has been your default for some time, is not a good reason to engage in sex. This behavior will lead to resentment, and your sexual satisfaction and feelings in the relationship will tank. If you are having sex only to avoid a negative outcome, you likely need to explore the option of couples therapy.

Alternatively, your sexual response cycle might be blocked because the stimuli you are exposed to are simply not working. Sometimes people engage in the same activity over and over throughout their lives, even if that activity no longer gives them pleasure. For example, perhaps in an earlier stage of your life you were aroused by your nipples being stimulated, but that no longer works for you. Perhaps you now find it painful, or you just don't feel anything. Repeated attempts to stimulate your nipples might leave you feeling frustrated. Sometimes the block in your sexual response cycle can occur because you are distracted and your brain is unable to process the incoming information and produce sexual arousal. Are you focused on how the sex will go? Are you worried that you might feel pain or that you might not become aroused? Are you concerned about how your partner might feel? When we are more attuned to the possible outcome of the sexual encounter than to the sensations in the moment, arousal (and orgasm) can be blocked. The good news is that mindfulness can help with this.

HOW MINDFULNESS CAN MEND THE BREAKS IN THE SEXUAL RESPONSE CYCLE

Mindfulness can help provide the skills you need to relate differently to breaks in the sexual response cycle. There is good scientific evidence that mindfulness can improve your ability to remain in the present moment, including paying attention to sexual sensations. Since mindfulness is about paying attention compassionately and without judgment, this means not evaluating or judging your sexual sensations but simply noticing them and allowing your mind and body to connect and respond with sexual arousal.

Being mindful might also help you pay attention to your own reasons for having sex and perhaps even discover reasons you weren't aware of. Re-read your own reasons for having sex and let the words be without thinking about them or reacting to them. This is mindfulness too. We will consider a much longer list of reasons for sex in chapter 8.

Paying attention to how your body responds to stimulation—whether it is physical touch, visual erotic triggers, sounds, or smells—is also amplified by mindfulness. Tuning in to a physical sensation that has been elicited by one of these triggers can lead to more intense sensations. In turn, the heightened sensations can invite you to pay even closer attention, which can lead to further heightened sensations. And so on.

When we tested this idea years ago with a group of gynecologic cancer survivors who stated that after their surgeries they "felt nothing" when their bodies were touched, we found that mindfulness taught them how to notice even the smallest physical sensations in their body. With practice, they learned how to remain with those sensations and to guide their attention back to those sensations when they became distracted or lost in their thoughts. After three months of mindfulness practice, they reported a significantly enhanced ability to notice arousal in their bodies. In some ways, mindfulness allows us to take a small sensation and make it much bigger.

It turns out that mindfulness is also helpful at the end of a sexual encounter. Earlier we discussed how a rewarding outcome of a sexual encounter can act as a motivation for future sexual encounters. If you evaluate the outcome as "terrible" or "unsatisfying," though, you are not likely to want to engage in sex in the future. Mindfulness can be a tool to allow you to observe the outcomes of a sexual encounter with less judgment and perhaps experience it as it is without evaluating it. Mindfulness also allows you to view thoughts such as "I should have responded more" or "I should have had an orgasm" as just mental events to be observed. Not truths. Not facts. And not predictions of how things will go in the future.

In sum, mindfulness is critical for your sexual response cycle. It is a part of feeling responsive sexual desire.

GETTING TO KNOW YOURSELF

The vulva and vagina are like snowflakes: no two are alike. They can also look different over time. Aging, birthing, hormonal changes, and health issues can lead to changes in the vulvovaginal tissues in a variety of ways. If you have never looked at yourself there, these changes might not be noticeable to you. Some of the ways that the vulva and vagina can change in appearance include the following:

· They can change in color, becoming paler or even losing their color altogether.
· They can become less plump.
· They can become less moist and soft.
· They can become thinner or more paperlike.
· The small lips (labia minora) may be less pronounced than in the past.
· There may be more skin or tissue covering the clitoris.

The following exercise provides a foundation for a series of body exploration exercises in later chapters that bridge your mindfulness practice with exploration of your body. As best you can, try to let go of any expectations about what this exercise will be like, even if you have looked at your genitals in this way before. I will elaborate a bit more on the characteristics of the vulva (including the clitoris) and the vagina in the next two sections. Note that these body parts are not one and the same, even though these terms are frequently and mistakenly used interchangeably.

Try to reserve about ten to fifteen minutes for this exercise. Try also to plan it at a time when there are few distractions and you are less likely to be interrupted. You can use a personal lubricant to minimize friction and feel more comfortable if you like.

Settle into a comfortable position (e.g., propped up against some pillows on your bed). Using a hand-held mirror, look at your genitals. You can consult the image below to see if you can find the parallel structure on yourself. I will guide you through reading about and then observing the clitoris and then the vagina.

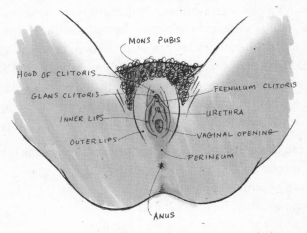

Illustration by Solita Work, Presence Creative © 2021

THE CLITORIS: MORE OF A COMPLEX THAN A BUTTON

The clitoris is quite a wonderful structure with no known function other than to give pleasure. It is formed of highly vascular tissue (i.e., dense with blood vessels) and is far more extensive than you might expect. If you look at the diagram, you will see the parts of the clitoris labeled "frenulum" (where the inner lips join the clitoris) and "glans" (which means head). These parts lie under the hood of the clitoris, which is a small fold of skin. The meaning of the word *clitoris* is unclear. Some sources suggest "little hill," others, "something that tickles," but I like the suggestion that it comes from *kleitors*, a Greek word meaning "divine and goddess-like."

The clitoris is far more elaborate and complex than most people realize. In addition to the frenulum and glans, it includes the *shaft* and *crura*, or legs, which are not visible in the image as they lie below the surface. Inside the shaft are two columns of spongy tissue called the *corpora cavernosa* (which literally means "cave-like body" and is not visible from the outside). As you become sexually stimulated and aroused, the corpora cavernosa fills with blood and increases the size of the clitoris. The shaft is usually between one and two inches long and half an inch wide but it may be smaller or larger. Once the shaft reaches the pubic bone it divides into the two crura, each of which can measure up to four inches long.

The crura are attached to and follow the arch of the pubic bone. There is even more clitoral tissue on each side of the vaginal opening toward the front and lying deep into the inner labia. These extensions are known as the *bulbs* of the clitoris. They are composed of the same spongy tissue and similarly swell with blood. Because they are much deeper, firmer massaging is needed to stimulate them to feel sexual pleasure, whereas the head of the clitoris, being on the surface, is highly sensitive. In fact, many women prefer not to be directly touched there with a finger or tongue unless they are sexually aroused.

The size of the clitoris varies greatly from one woman to the next, and its size does not predict the strength of an orgasm, or if a woman will even have an orgasm. Your own clitoris may protrude from the hood or be very hidden so that even when you pull back the clitoral hood, only a tiny amount of the clitoris is visible to you. When you stimulate yourself, the clitoris will enlarge and be much easier for you to feel.

Many women find out by accident, often in childhood, how they like the clitoris to be touched. Others deliberately set out to experiment in their teens or later. If you are uncertain about how you like to be stimulated and would like to experiment with touch, try stroking the length of the clitoris or gently massaging it with your fingertips in a circular motion. It may be that placing your whole hand over the clitoris and mons is more pleasurable for you, gently massaging with your whole hand and possibly pressing your middle finger down more directly onto the clitoris as you become more aroused. Exploring what feels good on your own helps you guide your partner when you are together. Try to bring mindful awareness as you examine your own clitoris, paying attention to colors, shape, texture, feelings of warmth, vibration, tension, and any other sensations that arise in you as you look and touch.

If you want to become even more "cliterate," I highly recommend the book *Becoming Cliterate*, written by my colleague Dr. Laurie Mintz.

THE VAGINA: A ROSE BY ANY OTHER NAME

The vagina is a tube of soft muscular tissue about three to five inches long. In a resting state, the walls of the vagina touch one another. This is surprising to some women who believe that the vagina is an open tube all the time. During sexual arousal, the vagina lengthens and stretches to accommodate a penis or dildo, and during childbirth it stretches to accommodate the passage of a baby. Some areas within the vagina may respond to sexual stimulation, but if yours does not, that is perfectly fine. The Grafenberg spot (the infamous G-spot) is an area located in the anterior wall of the vagina, less than two inches from the opening. Some women report experiencing very pleasurable sensations when this area is stimulated, say, by a finger, penis, or dildo. Not all women feel this sensitivity, however.

In some cultures, women's genitals are honored with wonderfully creative terms. In India and Tibet, for instance, they have been called at various points in time the "bell," "cup," "lotus flower" or "lotus of her wisdom," "pleasure filled of heaven," and "seat of pleasure." Over the centuries, the Chinese came up with dozens of names for the vagina, including the "door of life," "golden doorway," "golden furrow," "inner heart," "jade gate," "love grotto," "mysterious belly," and "perfumed mouth."

Unfortunately, in contrast to these beautiful and colorful names, many western countries refer to the vagina in derogatory terms such as "beaver," "pussy," or "hole," or even more negative terms. School sex education programs even fail to provide education on actual anatomical terms for the female anatomy, and instead use euphemisms like "privates" or "down there."

As you look at your own vagina during this exercise, try to bring a mindful self-compassion to observing it. If those names or labels come into your awareness, just treat them as mental events—perhaps descriptions you have come across in the past. They can float by as you continue to observe. Try to set aside these and other labels while you observe colors, textures, shapes, sizes, and sensations.

Try this self-awareness exercise a few times over the next week. Write your observations in your journal, noting the date and time of each practice.

STRUGGLES AND STRATEGIES

The struggles covered below pertain to the stretch and breath mindfulness practice, the sexual response cycle, and the exercise of observing your own vulva and vagina. I hope you find some of the strategies useful. If not, try to come up with your own!

THE STRUGGLE: FEELING TOO MUCH DISCOMFORT WITH THE
MINDFUL MOVEMENT PRACTICE

The mindful movement practice invites you to hold certain pos-
tures for an extended period while observing the sensations that
arise. You might find the sensations too intense to hold for the
length of time that the recording (or the written instruction)
specifies.

Strategies

· Try to tune in to the bare sensations and not focus on labeling
  an area as a source of pain. Sometimes when we label something
  as painful, the pain feels a lot less bearable. Instead, describe the
  feelings, using the sensations of pressure, temperature, texture,
  vibrations, location, and intensity to move closer to the actual
  feelings in a particular spot.

· If the intensity is too strong to bear, you can relax your body and
  stand (or sit) in stillness for a few moments before you resume
  the next movement.

· Be sure to cultivate lots of compassion toward yourself, no matter how easy, neutral, or difficult you find this practice.

THE STRUGGLE: THE SEXUAL RESPONSE CYCLE SEEMS TO
REQUIRE ME TO DO TOO MUCH TO CULTIVATE MY OWN
DESIRE.

It is true that in the sexual response cycle, sexual response,
arousal, and desire are very much under your control. This means
that what you do during a sexual encounter can have a direct
bearing on whether a sexual response unfolds or not. This might
feel like too much pressure on you while ignoring the influence
your partner might have on whether you feel arousal and desire.

Strategies

· Read this section a few times. We have been conditioned to
  believe that desire should just "happen" and that it is a necessary

precursor to sexual behavior and arousal. This is not true, and there is considerable scientific evidence that (1) arousal triggers desire and (2) you can engage in sexual activity even without desire, as long as you have reasons for having sex, and that desire can emerge during the encounter.

· Remember that because sexual desire is responsive, it can be influenced by you, your partner, and your environment. It is an empowering feeling to cultivate your own sexual desire.

· Break the sexual response cycle down into stages. Start by contemplating your own reasons for sexual activity and consider spending some time "trying on" different reasons for sex. Then focus on exploring the sexual stimuli that elicit arousal for you for a few weeks (or months). Be patient as you learn. You might feel embarrassed about examining your own body and using your hands to touch and explore. Don't worry. I will guide you through this in more detail in the sections ahead. Then move on to integrating the mindfulness skills that you are developing every day into your own sexual activity. Remember that this practice is simple but not easy.

THE STRUGGLE: I FEEL AWKWARD, EMBARRASSED, OR INHIBITED DURING THE MIRROR EXERCISE.
As I mentioned earlier, most women have never viewed their own genitals with a hand-held mirror. It is common to feel somewhat uncomfortable doing this.

Strategies

· Read the exercise over a few times and examine the diagram before trying it on your own.

· Be patient. Be kind. Try to observe mindfully and leave judgments aside.

TIME TO PRACTICE

Over the next week, try to do the mindful movement practice every second day. You can do the Body Scan on alternate days. As you practice, feel free to either use the audio recording or read the instructions in this chapter. Use your journal to track the date and time of your practice, and make notes about the sensations you observed.

Your informal mindfulness practice this week will be to pay more attention as you walk throughout your day. As in the Mindful Movement practice, see if you can notice sensations as you are walking that are pleasant, unpleasant, or neutral. You are not trying to change those sensations; rather, you are simply bringing awareness to them. Instead of specifying a length of time to spend on this, I suggest that you do this on at least one walk per day for however long works for you.

You might wish to read the information about the sexual response cycle a few times. You might also wish to read it, or paraphrase it, to a partner. If you do, what was their response?

The exercise of viewing your own genitals using a mirror could be done once a week, starting this week. Remember to find a time when you feel relaxed, when you have privacy, and where you have enough space and light to take your time.

4
Thoughts as Mental Sensations

A DIFFERENT WAY OF
THINKING ABOUT THOUGHTS

The mindfulness practice in this chapter involves mindfully noticing thoughts, which can be challenging, so I will discuss it first so that you have a stronger understanding of what it involves.

The mindfulness practices in the earlier chapters focused on tangible sensations—the sensations associated with food, with the various parts of the body, and with the breath. In this chapter we will still focus on "sensations," but instead of physical sensations, we will notice thoughts, which I will refer to as *mental sensations*. This helps reinforce that just as your body produces sensations (that are physical), your mind also produces sensations (that are mental). I will ask you to observe your mental sensations with the same openness, attention, and nonjudgment with which you observe your physical sensations. We also sometimes refer to these in the actual meditation as *mental events*.

Together we will *observe* thoughts rather than engaging in or following the content of them. This means that you have to be aware of when you are engaging in the content of thinking and to be able to alter how you are paying attention so that you can observe your thoughts without attachment. This is also known as *metacognition*, or watching yourself thinking. If it helps, imagine watching yourself think from a distance.

You will not empty your mind or suppress your thoughts. Nor will you try to modify your thoughts in any way. Many people misunderstand the instructions and make the mistake of believing that mindfulness requires them to shut off their thinking or their feelings. They somehow hear the instructions as meaning that a "good meditation" is one in which there is little or no thinking.

This is not true. Thinking is not bad or even undesirable during mindfulness practice. What matters is whether you are aware of your thoughts and feelings during meditation and how you handle them. Trying to suppress them may result in greater tension in your body and frustration in your mind. Mindfulness does not involve pushing thoughts away or closing yourself off from them to quiet your mind. You are not trying to stop your thoughts as they cascade through your mind. You are simply making room for them. This means learning how to observe them just as mental events and letting them be with an attitude of curiosity and acceptance.

FORMAL EXERCISE 4:
MINDFULNESS OF THOUGHTS PRACTICE

As you bring mindfulness to your thoughts in the following practice, you might notice that thoughts can be fleeting. Just when you notice them, they can disappear! Like all sensations we experience, thoughts are impermanent. You might also notice that some thoughts feel unpleasant and some feel pleasant. This Mindfulness of Thoughts practice will allow you to watch any habitual reaction you may have to push unpleasant thoughts away or to gravitate toward only pleasant thoughts and can help you avoid getting caught up in thoughts. Other thoughts feel neither pleasant nor unpleasant. They are simply neutral. Noticing a habitual reaction to seek out thoughts that are more "interesting" can make us more aware of when we drift off or our mind wanders—a nearly universal phenomenon!

In the practice that follows, try to notice your thoughts simply as mental events—a by-product of brain activity. In the same way that our skin produces billions of new cells each day, our brain produces mental sensations. Imagine if you had the same reaction to your thoughts as you do to the daily shedding of skin cells. I want you to bring the same curious but unattached attitude to thoughts as you do to other bodily processes. When we experience thoughts in this way, they begin to lose their dominance and importance and can be experienced as having the same level of significance as any other sensations, such as the physical sensations of the abdomen stretching during an inhale. Even especially negative or emotion-filled thoughts can lose their power and influence over us when we view them as "just something the brain does."

In *Full Catastrophe Living*, Kabat-Zinn suggests that we imagine ourselves sitting on the bank of a stream, firmly in place, resisting the temptation to get swept into the water. As we look down at the water in the stream, we see it moving by quickly. The stream represents our thoughts (you might have heard the term "stream of consciousness" applied to thoughts—and if you're an English grad, note that the term is not used in the same way as it is in literature). As we sit on the bank of the stream, we can watch the stream of water (i.e., our thoughts) go by, and we can watch those thoughts from a distance without getting caught up in their content.

If you take a step into the stream, you might get swept away by the content of your thoughts. When that happens, you might say to yourself, "I'm wet!" This is a crucial point. In that moment when you realize that you have become caught up in the content of the stream of thoughts, you can gently observe the content and qualities of that particular thought and then return your attention to observing the process of thinking, or, in this analogy, the flow of the stream. In that brief moment of getting caught up in the thought, you might worry that you're now lost in thoughts and that you won't be able to return to mindfully observing your thoughts from a distance. There is no need to worry. We all get swept up in thoughts. However, your ability to notice this "getting swept up" and then bring your awareness back to your body, or back to observing thoughts from a distance, will guide the development of your mindfulness skills.

When you remain planted on the bank of the stream, you can watch your thoughts go by. You might even categorize them as worrying thoughts, planning thoughts, happy thoughts, and so on.

If this analogy is helpful to you, use it in the Mindfulness of Thoughts practice that follows. Some people like to use other analogies, such as seeing clouds in the sky, with the gently moving clouds representing their thoughts. Others prefer to use the image of a train, with each of the boxcars representing a thought. As you stand at the side of the railway track, you can watch these thoughts (the boxcars) passing by, without jumping on the train. Whatever analogy you choose, remember that it is meant to be a helpful way of relating to thoughts as mental events that can be experienced from a distance. If using an analogy does not work for you, that is fine too. Just follow the instructions below without imagining the thoughts as a stream (or clouds or boxcars).

WHAT YOU WILL NEED

- A chair, ideally high-back
- A quiet space (remember that no space will be totally silent, and that is okay!)
- Comfortable socks or shoes
- Your journal

This practice will take about twenty minutes.

STEP-BY-STEP GUIDE TO MINDFULNESS OF THOUGHTS

- Start by settling into a comfortable sitting position. Take the time now to make any adjustments so you are sitting as comfortably as you can in an upright and dignified posture. Check to see that your spine, neck, and head are in alignment and your feet are flat on the floor. Let your hands rest on your thighs or in your lap. Allow your eyes to gently close if this feels comfortable, or, if you prefer, you can choose a spot in front of you and focus on it with a soft gaze.

- Settle into the sensations of sitting, just as you find them, right here, right now. Allow your attention to move fluidly from sensation to sensation, as each arises and fades in prominence.

- Do your best to stay alert and mentally focused throughout the practice.

- When you are ready, move your focus of attention from the sensations of your body sitting here to focus more narrowly on the sensations of breathing. Become aware of each in-breath and each out-breath as they follow, one after the other.

- Whenever you notice that your attention has moved to a physical sensation elsewhere in your body, a sound, or a thought that is more predominant, momentarily take this to be the new focus of attention. When it is no longer predominant, bring the focus of your attention back to the sensations of breathing.

- In this practice, it is often helpful to follow your breath in one part of your body. There may be a number of places in your body where your breath makes itself known. Focus your attention now on the patterns of physical sensations, beginning at your nostrils, as your breath moves into and out of your body. As you breathe in, feel the sensations at your nostrils as the cooler air is drawn into your body. And then, on the out-breath, feel the sensations of friction or pressure at your nostrils as the warm air leaves your body. You do not need to breathe in any particular way or use your breath to get anywhere. Just let your breath be there as it is.

- When you are ready, move the focus of your attention down your body to your chest and notice the sensations in this area. Feel the expansion of your chest as you breathe in, and the falling away of your chest as you breathe out. Tune in to this gentle rhythm of your chest's rising and falling as you breathe. Observe the sensations of breathing in this part of your body.

- Now, when you are ready, move the focus of your attention farther down your body to your abdomen and belly. Feel the expansion of your belly as it rises on the in-breath and the gentle deflation of your belly on the out-breath. As best as you can, focus as closely as possible on your breath as it enters your body on the in-breath, and all the way through as it leaves your body on the out-breath. Perhaps notice the slight pauses between one in-breath and the following out-breath, and between one out-breath and the following in-breath.

- You may choose to stay with the breath at your belly, or you may choose another place where your breath makes itself known to you most vividly and stay with that as the primary focus of your attention.

- Whenever you notice that you have forgotten about noticing your breath sensations because your attention was engaged with a thought, congratulate yourself for becoming aware of that. This is perfectly okay. It's simply what our minds do. It doesn't mean you've made a mistake or that you're doing anything wrong. Notice what your attention was engaged with and then, with compassion, return your attention to the sensations of breathing in the region you are focusing on. Even if your attention becomes engaged in thoughts many times during this mindfulness practice, simply notice this and return your attention over and over again to the sensations of breathing, without any judgment or blame, and just start over again. Use your breath as an anchor to gently reconnect with the here-and-now.

· When you are ready, you can expand the field of your awareness to include your entire body, from the top of your head to the soles of your feet. Pay careful attention to the many individual sensations that arise and pass away within this larger field of your awareness, wherever those sensations may be located in your body. Allow your attention to move fluidly from sensation to sensation, wherever they are arising in your body, focusing for a moment on each one, as it rises and fades in prominence. Without too much straining, try to observe each sensation as clearly as possible, just as it is. Perhaps notice the sensations where your body makes contact with the floor or the chair. And bring a friendly, interested attention to the sensations of touch or pressure. Can you feel sensations in your buttocks where they make contact with the chair? Can you notice sensations in your hands where they rest on your thighs or on each other? Perhaps notice the sensations of breathing at your nostrils, chest, or belly.

· When you engage in a mindfulness practice for some time like this, it is not unusual for strong sensations to emerge. You may feel discomfort, pain, or tension and find that your attention is repeatedly drawn to these sensations. There are a couple of ways of working with such sensations. One way is to simply move or adjust your body. If you choose to do this, try to form an intention to move before you actually move. Then notice the sensations of moving and the sensations following your movement. In this way, your response to strong sensations can be guided by the same principles of choice and awareness that you have been practicing all along.

- The other way of working with strong sensations is to bring your attention right up to—or even into—the region of intensity itself. While your awareness is there, try to greet what you find there with an attitude of openness and curiosity. As best as you can, observe with gentle and wise attention the detailed pattern of sensations you find there. Ask yourself, "What do these sensations feel like? Where exactly are they? Do they change over time or move from one part of my body to another? What smaller sensations do I notice inside the general sense of the strong sensation?" Make the strong sensations the focus of your attention for as long as they are predominant.

- If you notice that your attention has become engaged in the content of a thought or perhaps has moved to a memory triggered by that thought, you can always return your attention to the present moment by refocusing on the movements of your breath. Then you can choose whether to stay with your breath as the focus of attention or to return to observing the strong sensations in your body. And if the intensity of these sensations fades, you can allow your attention to move fluidly from sensation to sensation throughout the body as each rises and fades in prominence.

- Now gently move the focus of your attention from the sensations of your body to the sensations of sound. Bring your attention to your ears and then allow your awareness to open and expand so that you are receptive to sounds as they arise, wherever they are.

- There is no need to go searching for sounds or to listen for particular sounds. Instead, as best as you can, simply open your awareness so that it is receptive to sounds from all directions as they arise—sounds that are close, sounds that are far away, sounds that are in front, behind, to the side, above, or below you.

Open your ears to all of the sounds around you now. Become aware of both obvious and more subtle sounds, of the space between sounds, and even of silence.

- As best as you can, become aware of sounds simply as sensations. Whenever you find that you are thinking about the sounds, reconnect, as best you can, with awareness of their sensory qualities, such as their patterns of pitch, timbre, loudness, and duration, rather than their meanings or implications.

- Whenever you notice that your attention has moved from sounds to a physical sensation in your body or to a thought that has become predominant, momentarily take this to be the new focus for your attention and bring the same level of mindful awareness to that sensation, or thought, continuing to observe it until it is no longer predominant. Then bring your attention back to sounds.

- Whenever you notice that you have forgotten about noticing sounds because your attention was engaged in or wrapped up in the content of a thought, congratulate yourself on becoming aware of that. Notice what your attention had been engaged with and then, with gentle compassion, return your attention to sounds.

- When you are ready, let go of sounds as the focus of your attention and focus your attention on thoughts as events in your mind. You can do the same with thoughts as you did with sounds: notice them arise, develop, and pass away. As best as you can, bring awareness to thoughts that arise in your mind by noticing when thoughts arise and focusing your awareness on them as they pass through the space of the mind and eventually disappear. There is no need to try to make thoughts come or go. Just let them arise naturally, in the same way that you responded to sounds arising and fading away.

- Some people find it helpful to bring awareness to thoughts in their mind in the same way that they might if the thoughts were projected on the screen at a movie theater. You sit watching the screen, waiting for a thought or image to arise. When it does, you pay attention to it for as long as it is there on the screen and then you let it go as it passes away. If this imagery works for you, stay with it. Alternatively, you may find it helpful to see thoughts as clouds moving across a vast, spacious sky, or as a stream of water passing by, or even as the boxcars of a passing train.

- If any thoughts bring with them intense feelings or emotions, pleasant or unpleasant, try, as best as you can, to just observe any "emotional charge" and intensity associated with them, as you allow them to be as they are.

- If at any time you feel that your attention has become unfocused and scattered, or if it keeps getting repeatedly drawn into the story of your thinking or imagining, you may want to notice where this is affecting your body. Often, when we don't like what is happening, we feel a sense of contraction or tightness in the face, shoulders, or torso and a sense of wanting to push away our thoughts and feelings. Notice if any of this is going on for you when intense feelings arise. Once you have noticed this, come back to the sensations of breathing and use this focus to anchor and stabilize your awareness.

- Continue to observe your thoughts from a distance for a few more minutes. As you are observing thoughts from a distance, take note of whether there is any liking or disliking of them.

- At a certain point, when it feels right to you, let go of any particular object of attention, like your breath or thoughts or sounds, and just allow your field of awareness to be open to whatever arises in the landscape of your mind and body. Simply rest in awareness, effortlessly being aware of whatever arises from moment to moment. That might include your breath, sensations in your body, sounds, thoughts, or feelings. As best you can, just sit, completely awake, not holding on to anything, not looking for anything, having no agenda other than embodied wakefulness.

- Whenever you're ready, allow your eyes to open if they were closed. If your eyes were open, raise your gaze now directly in front of you. Shift the focus from sensations in your body to a deeper reflection on your experience and how it relates to sexuality.

- Finally, take a few deep breaths before you move on to the Inquiry.

THE INQUIRY

By now you will be familiar with the three questions posed in the Inquiry. Because you have focused on thoughts during this mindfulness practice, however, your observations might be quite different from your earlier ones. As always, there is no right or wrong answer to these questions. Instead, I invite you to tune in to yourself, without filters or judgment, to see what arises. Consider writing the answers to these questions in your journal. Otherwise, simply take time to think about them.

QUESTION 1. What did you notice during this practice when you were invited to pay attention to sounds and thoughts?

How did you find this practice of mindfully noticing sounds and thoughts? Could you watch yourself thinking? What kinds of mental sensations (thoughts) did you notice? If you were swept away by the content of your thoughts—as many people are—at what point did you notice? What did you do next? Could you haul yourself out of the stream (using the analogy of thoughts as a stream of water) and return to the bank, where you could once again watch your thoughts from a distance? Could you channel compassion toward yourself when this happened?

Once you settled into observing your thoughts from a distance, what did you notice about them? Did you experience your thoughts as temporary or transient? Was there any pattern or predictability to the kinds of thoughts you had?

Where did you perceive the thoughts as occurring? Were they inside your body? Outside your body? Could you pinpoint a precise location either within or outside the body where the thought seemed to occur? Did different thoughts occur in different locations?

Did your thoughts vary in size and intensity? How did you know when a thought was big or small? Did they have any visual component? Were the thoughts associated with hearing, smelling, or tasting?

How long did a thought typically last? Did some thoughts last longer than others? If you perceived a thought primarily through sound, could you perceive any of the individual sounds that made up the thought? If so, were you able to perceive the beginning and end of each syllable? If a thought had a visual component, could you sense whether the image was in black and white or color? How large was the image? Was it clear or fuzzy? Could you see the edges of the image? Did the image seem to flash or flicker? If the thought had a physical component (such as the memory of a physical sensation), were you able to perceive the individual sensations that made up the physical memory?

QUESTION 2. How was paying attention to your thoughts in this way different from how you normally experience thoughts in your life?

Now that you have tuned in to the sensations that emerged as you tried to observe thoughts, consider how this process of watching thoughts from a distance is different from how you normally engage with thoughts in your life. Have you ever deliberately kept this distance from your thoughts as you were having them?

QUESTION 3. How was this Mindfulness of Thoughts exercise relevant to your sexuality?

You have just explored the characteristics of mental events and considered how observing them in this way is different from how you normally experience thoughts. In what ways might this be relevant to your sexuality or your experiences of sexual difficulties? Could this skill of watching thoughts as though they are streams of water passing before you, without becoming attached to any of them, be helpful in the event that you experience negative judgments about your own sexuality? Could this skill be used during a sexual encounter when you find yourself lost in thoughts? Or when you notice that you are spending more time worrying about the outcome of a sexual encounter than actually participating in the act of sex itself?

END OF THE MINDFULNESS OF THOUGHTS PRACTICE
Congratulations on finishing the Mindfulness of Thoughts practice and the Inquiry. You might wish to stand and move around before continuing.

The hundreds of women who have participated in our face-to-face mindful sex program have often noted that they find this mindfulness practice one of the more challenging we introduce them to. Because many of them have spent a lifetime being a slave to their own thoughts, the process of creating space between them and their thoughts can feel strange. If as soon as you notice a thought it magnetically draws you into it, leading you to follow it, then moving you quickly to the next thought, and the next one after that, it can be very hard to remain firmly planted at the side of the stream watching your thoughts go by. But don't interpret any challenges you encounter with this practice as a sign that you're not capable of creating distance between you and your thoughts. This might be an entirely new way of relating to your thoughts—it certainly is for most of the women in our groups—and will take practice before you become comfortable with it.

Here are some of the observations women in our groups have made:

- When I noticed the first thought, it was lightning speed before the next one came and the next one after that. I was surprised to see how quickly a single thought could take me to so many more.

- When I pushed myself to look at thoughts as "mental events," I noticed that they had certain qualities to them, in the same way that I discovered by observing my breath that it had certain physical qualities to it. For example, most of my mental events were memories of past events as opposed to thoughts about the present moment or about the future. Bringing attention to the specific qualities of my thoughts was quite helpful to notice that.

- I noticed that when I was having negative thoughts during the practice my body would stiffen up and my face would wrinkle. I never knew that thoughts could affect my body so strongly!

- I noticed that my mind really does produce random thoughts that are not linked to each other! I can be thinking a hundred different things in a single minute!

- As soon as I noticed a thought and tried to observe it more clearly, it disappeared.

- I saw that I have a lot of thoughts about things I "should" be doing or not doing. Is this "shoulding myself in the foot"?

In between the noticeably positive thoughts and negative ones, I had a whole bunch of random and neutral thoughts that didn't lead me to feel any emotion. That was surprising to me as I thought that all thoughts were either good or bad. I hadn't considered that some thoughts can have no feelings associated with them.

In your mindfulness practice, you want to be in a place where all thoughts—positive, negative, and neutral—can be observed as sensations that arise and pass away, without making any attempt to suppress, judge, or in any other way engage in their content. This can be a difficult exercise, but repeated practice and experience with treating thoughts as mental events will make this easier. Try to consider the idea that even thoughts with a very unpleasant feeling, tone, and content that many of us might categorize as "negative" are in fact transient mental events, brain sensations, and not necessarily truths. Accepting that thoughts such as this arise from time to time but then choosing not to follow them or engage in their content can lead to major changes in how you experience emotions and sensations, including those related to sexual activity.

HOW MIGHT MINDFULNESS OF THOUGHTS IMPROVE ASPECTS OF SEXUALITY?

As you pay attention to your moment-to-moment experience during mindfulness practice, you might have noticed that you can be bombarded with a seemingly never-ending stream of thoughts coming out of the blue in rapid succession. Many people are greatly relieved to discover that they are not the only ones whose thoughts cascade through their mind like a waterfall. But how might this observation benefit your sexuality?

When you have a thought about yourself sexually, especially if it is a negative one—for example, "I will never be able to have an orgasm"—it can feel like this thought defines you. Or, by virtue of having the thought, you might be more inclined to believe that it is true. ("If this thought were not true, then why would I be feeling this way?") If you are in a period of high stress, your mind will tend to obsess about your predicament, what you should do or should have done, or what you shouldn't do or shouldn't have done. At such times your thoughts might be highly charged with anxiety and worry. But remember: you are not your thoughts. In this practice, you are relating to your thoughts as sensations just like any other sensation. In experiencing your thoughts in this way, you might learn that thoughts change from moment to moment, that some are pleasant and others are unpleasant, and that you are not defined by your thoughts.

For many people this discovery is a revelation, and it can set the stage for a profound learning experience that many claim is the most valuable thing they get out of their mindfulness training: the realization that they are not their thoughts. This discovery means that when you have negative thoughts about your sexuality, you can consciously choose to relate or not to relate to those thoughts in a variety of ways that were not available to you when you were unaware of this simple fact.

In addition to negative or judgmental thoughts you might have about yourself and your sexuality, you might also experience a large number of benign or neutral thoughts—but those thoughts also interfere with your sexual response. Sometimes they can dominate your attention during sex and make you forget what you are doing. At less stressful times, the thoughts that go through your mind might be more benign, but their content can be just as enticing. You might find yourself thinking about a movie you saw, or about dinner, work, your parents or your children, an upcoming vacation, your health, death, your bills...

Mindful awareness of your thoughts can help you stay connected to the sexual experience and be less swept away by thoughts about the way things have been or will be rather than the way they are in this moment, or by planning for events in your future, many of which you will have no control over. Remember the sexual response cycle in chapter 3? Thoughts during sex have a way of interfering with your attention, which can disrupt the cycle that leads to sexual arousal and desire. By observing your thoughts mindfully and simply as mental events, you allow the sexual response cycle to flow naturally so that sexual triggers can elicit your arousal and desire. In other words, mindfully observing thoughts promotes a healthy sexual response cycle in which a combination of your initial reasons for sex and effective sexual triggers can lead to sexual arousal and desire.

EDUCATION ABOUT SEX: BELIEFS AND OTHER THOUGHTS

SEXUAL BELIEFS

Thoughts that arise during sex, especially those that are negative or judgmental, might be the by-product of deeply held beliefs about sex that you developed via explicit or implicit societal or cultural messages you heard from your family, community, or religion. While sexual beliefs might certainly be based on truth or reality, sometimes—often!—they are not. And when they are not, they can negatively affect your sexual experience, the way you view sexuality, and your sexual esteem.

Remember the Four P's—predisposing, precipitating, perpetuating, and protective factors—from chapter 2? Early life experiences or teachings can predispose you to have certain beliefs about sex, or about yourself as a sexual person, when you are an adult. Although the seeds of those beliefs might have been sown when you were a child, the fruits of their influence ripen during your day-to-day sexual experiences.

The Mindfulness of Thoughts practice you just completed might have illuminated some of your thoughts about sex.

Mindfulness offers a practical way of relating to these thoughts purely as mental events, but it can also help you understand the roots of such thoughts. To do that, you first need to consider your own sexual beliefs. Think about the following questions and observations:

· What role do you think your sexual beliefs might have played in your experience of sexuality? Record your thoughts about this in your journal.

· What do you think sex *should* be? Here are some examples of what women in our mindful sex groups have said when we asked them to complete the sentence "Sex should":

  · come naturally.
  · be spontaneous or at least not scheduled.
  · include vaginal penetration or intercourse.
  · include orgasm and ideally a vaginal orgasm.
  · always be an expression of love.
  · always be an expression of lust.
  · start with sexual desire.

In your journal list some of your own beliefs that would complete the sentence "Sex should…"

· Now think about your own beliefs regarding what *you should* be or not be when it comes to sex. Here are some examples of what women who have participated in our program in the past said when we asked them to complete the sentence "I should":

  · not have sexual problems (they're for older people/for people who don't love their partners/for women who aren't confident).
  · not be assertive sexually (good girls don't do this).
  · know what I like sexually.
  · be able to communicate to a partner about sex.

In your journal list some of your own beliefs that would complete the sentence: "I should…"

· Finally, think about your beliefs about your partner and the *shoulds*. Do you have particular beliefs about what your partner should do or not do? What they should know or not know when it comes to sex? Here are some examples of what women who have participated in our program in the past said when we asked them to complete the sentence "My partner should":

  · know what I like/want, and the longer we have been together, the more they should know and I should not have to tell them.
  · have intercourse in order for sex to be satisfying.

In your journal list some of your own beliefs that would complete the sentence: "My partner should…"

TAKE A MOMENT to read what you wrote about what sex should be and what you and your partner should do regarding sex. Can you identify any feelings that come up? Are you aware of any sensations in your body as you re-read these shoulds? You might not be aware of when and how often certain sexual beliefs are activated. In fact, we often do not pay attention to such beliefs. But rigid beliefs can affect how we feel and our mood more generally, and we are often aware of emotions such as sadness, frustration, guilt, and anxiety around sex. Paying attention to sexual beliefs can help you understand what contributes to how you feel sexually.

One way to become more aware of your sexual beliefs is to pause and "check in" whenever you experience a strong emotion related to your sexuality. Maybe you see something (like a sex scene in a movie) that triggers this reaction, or perhaps a partner brings up a difficult subject related to sex or their dissatisfaction.

When this happens, try to tune in to how you are feeling in that moment. What emotion or set of emotions do you notice? How does this manifest in physical sensations? Now use the "sex should/I should/my partner should" format to help you see if you are aware of particular beliefs about sex. One reason that mindfulness is so effective in managing sexual difficulties is that it provides a tool for bringing awareness to what is already there. And once you are aware, acceptance is just a breath away.

COMMONLY HELD BELIEFS ABOUT WOMEN AND SEX

As you continue reading and working through this workbook, pause to reflect on any beliefs that come to the surface. You can ask yourself, "What am I thinking?" and tune in to physical sensations and emotions that arise as you bring awareness to your thoughts. Over time, you might notice a particular pattern to the kinds of sex-related beliefs you have. For example, many women have sex-related beliefs that stem from an underlying dissatisfaction with their own bodies. As a result, the following beliefs might arise :

· I can't have sex with the light on.

· I can't allow my partner to see my body shape.

· My weight prevents me from experiencing sexual arousal.

· My lack of physical fitness makes it impossible for me to sustain a certain position in sex long enough to have an orgasm.

These are just a few examples. There are countless more—unfortunately.

Consider the following beliefs. As you read each one, circle the number that corresponds to how strongly you believe it, from 0 (I do not believe it at all) to 10 (I completely believe this).

(1) Sex is only for young people.

0   1   2   3   4   5   6   7   8   9   10

(2) "Normal" women have an orgasm every time they have sex.

0   1   2   3   4   5   6   7   8   9   10

(3) A woman's sexual life ends with menopause.

0   1   2   3   4   5   6   7   8   9   10

(4) Only spontaneous sex is "good" sex.

0   1   2   3   4   5   6   7   8   9   10

(5) If you love your partner, sex will be wonderful.

0   1   2   3   4   5   6   7   8   9   10

(6) Sex should include vaginal penetration/intercourse and orgasm.

0   1   2   3   4   5   6   7   8   9   10

(7) Sex should start with sexual desire.

0   1   2   3   4   5   6   7   8   9   10

(8) My partner should know what I like/want, and the longer we have been together, the more they should know and I should not have to tell them.

0   1   2   3   4   5   6   7   8   9   10

(9) My partner's sexual needs come before my own sexual wants.

0   1   2   3   4   5   6   7   8   9   10

(10) Affectionate touching always leads to sex.

0   1   2   3   4   5   6   7   8   9   10

(11) No one has sexual problems except me.

0   1   2   3   4   5   6   7   8   9   10

(12) Sex should be easy.

0   1   2   3   4   5   6   7   8   9   10

(13) Only vaginal penetration is real sex. Everything else is "extra."

0　1　2　3　4　5　6　7　8　9　10

(14) Only vaginal orgasms are real orgasms.

0　1　2　3　4　5　6　7　8　9　10

(15) My partner needs to have vaginal penetration/intercourse for sex to be satisfying

0　1　2　3　4　5　6　7　8　9　10

Add up your total score. If it was higher than 0, you might have beliefs about sex that could be directly interfering with your sexual response and putting up a barrier between you and a satisfying sex life. If you did not endorse any of these beliefs, congratulations! But do you have other beliefs that are not on this list? If so, write them down in your journal. Writing them down enhances your awareness, and awareness is the gateway to change.

BODY IMAGE AND MINDFULNESS
You might argue that mindfulness is essentially a body-oriented practice, since you are using your awareness in a compassionate and nonjudgmental way to tune in to sensations in your body. But mindfulness can also be useful for how you see yourself.

Chapters 1 and 2 considered how negative body image can influence sexual difficulties. A repeated focus on how your body looks, in a negative and judgmental way, can interfere with all aspects of your sexual response, from desire to arousal to orgasm to satisfaction. According to the research, severe concerns about body image can predispose a person to sexual problems. As you saw in chapter 2, if you have a strong negative view of your body, it is difficult to have a sense of self-worth. Some people deliberately conceal their bodies during sexual activity by keeping the lights off or only having sex under the covers and with their eyes closed. Others extend this practice of hiding to other intimate activities—for example, avoiding undressing in front of a partner. When you conceal your body, you are effectively putting up a barrier between you and your partner. This limits opportunities for touching and nonsexual but intimate sharing between you.

Some of the women in our groups struggle during the Mindful Movement practice because the movements might have led them to scrutinize their bodies, especially if they felt that they were not doing the practice "well enough." For some women, the illustration of female genital anatomy also activated concerns about body image. In some of the exercises that follow I will ask you to engage in self-touching. This can elicit negative thoughts and feelings as well as tension in the body. Different women have different levels of comfort with these exercises, and mindfulness is one way of bringing some acceptance to your practice.

A MINDFUL APPROACH TO EASING NEGATIVE BODY IMAGE

Unfortunately, lingering societal taboos about women and masturbation sometimes compound existing body image issues. The purpose of this exercise—which was adapted from Julia Heiman and Joseph LoPiccolo's 1976 book, *Becoming Orgasmic: A Sexual Growth Program for Women*, one of the best self-help books about how to reach orgasm ever written—is to allow you to practice nonjudgmental awareness of your own naked body.

It uses the same nonjudgmental attention skills you have been practicing in the formal meditations so far and focuses on the sensations elicited during and after a bath or shower. It will take you about fifteen to thirty minutes to complete. If possible, do this exercise near a mirror, as the final instructions ask you to look at yourself in the mirror. Try to practice at a time when your mind is not flooded with thoughts! Read the instructions below in full before you start.

INFORMAL EXERCISE: FOCUSING PRACTICE

· Start by taking a bath or a shower. As you do so, try to notice particular parts of your body, such as your hands, arms, breasts, stomach, legs, and feet. Try to focus your attention on the visual attributes of your body (e.g., the texture of your skin, its color, crevices, ridges, smooth patches, etc.) and let your thoughts simply be as they are in the background.

· To enhance your experience, use all of your senses. Take note of all the smaller sensations that make up any larger ones.

· What sounds meet your ears as you wash? Close your eyes for a moment and tune in to the individual qualities of the sounds.

· Do the same for smells that emerge during your bath or shower. Observe also neutral smells or the absence of smells. Everything that arises in your attentional field is an opportunity for mindfulness.

· After you have finished showering or bathing, mindfully dry yourself, once again using all of your senses. Observe the transformation of your skin from wet to dry. Feel the towel fabric against your skin. Notice temperatures and changes in temperature.

· When mental events surface, acknowledge that they are there and then let them fade into the background.

· After you have dried yourself, spend a few minutes looking at yourself in a mirror. What can you appreciate about your body? (Think about function—not just appearance.)

· Are there parts of your body that give you a sense of pleasure or pride? Are there any parts of yourself that do not give you a sense of pleasure or pride?

· Tell yourself, "My body is alive." Close your eyes and tune in to any sensations that arise when you say this.

- Are there aspects of your body that deserve more attention? Perhaps there are parts of your body that you judge or dislike or even hate. Bring your mindful awareness to each of these parts in turn and try to observe the bare sensations without labeling them. As you do this, notice any emotions you may be feeling—both positive and negative. As you have done in previous chapters, notice any attachment to pleasant sensations and aversion to negative sensations. Welcome all the sensations that arrive.

- Still standing in front of the mirror with your eyes still closed, take a few moments to tune in to the sensations arising from inside your body.

- When you are ready, open your eyes. Look at your whole body in the mirror and take your whole self in.

Try to do this focusing exercise at least a few times over the next week, or perhaps even every time you have a bath or shower. Remember that the goal is not to change any thoughts you have about your body but to foster awareness and acceptance.

In your journal, write the date(s) on which you practiced this and any mental or physical sensations you noticed during the exercise.

SEX, MINDFULNESS, AND BODY IMAGE: A CONVERSATION WITH A FRIEND

In our mindful sex groups, we encourage participants to have a conversation with a trusted friend about body image and sexuality and how they are related. Sometimes the effects of a negative body image are so deeply ingrained that you might not even be aware of its effects on your sexuality. In such situations, talking about the body image–sex relationship can increase your awareness of your beliefs about body image, and this awareness itself can sometimes give rise to change.

If you have never talked to a trusted friend or family member about your sexuality, you might find this conversation challenging. One way to introduce it is to say something like "I heard something on the radio [or read something] that talked about how important it is to acknowledge sexual health as a part of quality of life and that for a lot of people body image is part of it. I wonder if you'd be open to talking about this with me." If this seems daunting, know that hundreds of women in our mindful sex groups have expressed discomfort with this exercise, convinced themselves that they could not have this conversation, and then in the end experienced it as "not that bad" and, in fact, quite valuable for shedding light on the many ways that their body image affects their sexuality. We offer some guidelines on how to initiate and carry out this conversation:

· Try to choose someone you feel comfortable discussing personal topics with. You might have had discussions about health, relationships, emotional issues, or even your sexuality with this person in the past.

· Share with one another how you define body image. What does it mean to you? And to your friend? This is a great way to ease into the conversation.

· Now you can move on to talking about the situations in which concerns about body image come up for you. Are there places, people, or activities that are more likely to activate negative thoughts or feelings about your body? What happens when such feelings are evoked? What do you do? You and your friend can take turns answering these questions.

· Next, consider how body image, as you've just defined it, affects your sexuality. Think broadly about your sexual beliefs, your desire, your arousal, your sexual satisfaction, your ability to communicate about sex, your distress about sex, and any other aspect of sexuality that might be affected by body image. Ask your friend this question as well.

· Take note of any feelings that come up for you (emotionally as well as physically) as you are having this conversation. Bring a mindful self-compassion to yourself no matter what arises.

Once the conversation is over, write down any observations you made in your journal. Were you surprised by what you said? Did talking about this with someone else give you any new insights into the role of your body image on your own sexuality? Did you learn anything from hearing your friend talk about their relationship between body image and sexuality? Now think about how you could use mindfulness to ease the effects of your body image on your sexuality. How might you use mindfulness to strengthen your body image and thus influence its effects on your sexuality?

INCORPORATING TOUCH

In chapter 3, I encouraged you to get to know your vulva. You may have used a mirror to observe your genitals, and you may have looked at the diagram of the vulva in that chapter. If you did not do either of these, I invite you to do so now, before moving on to the next practice, which introduces touch.

Touch is an important component of the sexual experience. In this exercise I will invite you to touch yourself with your fingers as a way of eliciting and feeling bare sensations as they arise in response to your self-touch. The purpose of this practice is to strengthen your awareness of your body—to remind you that parts of you that are important to your sexual experience are capable of giving you pleasure even if you have problems with sex or pain. You may have never taken part in explorative self-touching before, or perhaps you tried it once and never again.

During this exercise, you may experience negative emotions or thoughts that your sexual parts are foreign or unpleasant. You may feel uncomfortable about the very idea of touching yourself. This is to be expected, given our society's negative messages about women's genitals and women's sexuality more generally. Try to relate to these emotions and thoughts as mental events, something produced by your brain's activity, rather than as facts or statements of reality.

INFORMAL EXERCISE: SELF-OBSERVATION AND TOUCHING PRACTICE

Try to reserve about ten to fifteen minutes for this exercise. Plan it for a time when there are few distractions and you are not likely to be interrupted. Have your preferred nonirritating body lotion, oil, or powder, your personal lubricant, and a hand-held mirror in hand. You will find this exercise more comfortable if your fingernails are short. Remove your lower articles of clothing for easier access to yourself.

- Settle into a comfortable position (e.g., propped up against some pillows on your bed). Begin by closing your eyes and briefly checking in with your experience in this moment. Ask yourself, "How am I feeling right now? What sensations do I feel in my body right now? Am I aware of particular mental events right now, before I get started?"

- Slowly begin to explore your body with touch. Apply your body lotion, oil, or powder to your arms and legs. As you do so, keep your eyes closed so that you can focus your attention on those physical feelings of touch. Notice what different parts of your body feel like—the sensations of shape, temperature, and texture in your fingers and hands. Notice any and all the sensations produced in the area you are touching. Breathe.

- Whenever you notice that your attention is no longer on touch sensations, gently and kindly redirect it to those sensations in your fingers and hands and the area you are touching. Be kind to yourself if you find your attention wavering. Mindfulness is about noticing compassionately, including when you notice that your mind has gone elsewhere.

- After touching and bringing awareness to the feelings in your arms and legs, move your hands to your torso. Touch your abdomen, your chest, and your neck and face.

- After you have spent about ten minutes on these other parts of your body, move your hands to your genitals. Place your handheld mirror a few inches up from your vulva so you can observe the different structures. Start by paying attention to the colors, shapes, sizes, and areas of dark versus light. Bring your awareness to your thoughts and take note of any mental events that are active right now. Continue to pay attention to them while you observe your genitals.

- Next, notice if any emotions arise along with those thoughts. Do you notice any physical sensations as you are looking? Describe the sensations to yourself—for example, the textures, areas that are more moist than others, and temperature. Take time to notice what your genitals look like. Take a deep breath.

- When you are ready, press your fingers gently on the area of your clitoris, noticing how different amounts of pressure produce different sensations. Rub some lubricant on your fingers and then move your fingers down to touch the outer entrance of your vagina. When you are ready, move one or more fingers inside.

- Remind yourself that the goal of this exercise is not to become aroused or reach orgasm but to enhance your awareness of your body. Try to contract your vaginal muscles and notice what that feels like in your genitals and against your finger(s). As you do so, remind yourself that these areas play an important part in your sexual pleasure and experience.

· What thoughts or mental sensations are you aware of right now? Is there a feeling that accompanies the thoughts? Can you notice those mental sensations just as you observed the stream of water passing by while you remained firmly planted at a distance, on the shore? Just because thoughts are there does not mean you have to "run with them" and does not make them truths. If the mental sensations become stronger, notice if you feel any aversion to them or a desire to move away from them. If that happens, you can briefly stop touching yourself while you take three deep breaths. Then continue touching.

· After exploring sensations in your genitals for a few minutes, you may wish to end the exercise by moving your hands back to a non-genital area on your body. When you are finished, take note of any emotions or thoughts that arose during this exercise. If this session was disappointing for any reason, try to also acknowledge any aspects of the session that were positive or neutral. Each session will be different and will be a new opportunity to learn and explore.

Try this self-awareness exercise two or more times before you go on to chapter 5. In your journal, write the dates on which you practiced this and any thoughts, emotions, or physical sensations you noticed during the exercise.

INFORMAL EXERCISE:
THE 3-MINUTE BREATHING SPACE PRACTICE

The psychologists, researchers, and mindfulness experts John Teasdale, J. Mark Williams, and Zindel Segal, who developed mindfulness-based cognitive therapy, also developed a short mindfulness practice called the 3-Minute Breathing Space. This practice may be short but it includes all the key features of a longer mindfulness practice: bringing attention to the present moment, feeling self-compassion, focusing on physical sensations, and letting thoughts "be." That makes it a portable mindfulness practice that can be used essentially anywhere or anytime.

The three steps of the 3-Minute Breathing Space are wide focus, then narrow focus, then wide focus again. As the name implies, each step lasts one minute.

Step 1: Come into the moment.

- Adopt a relaxed, dignified posture with your back upright but not stiff, and let your body sense being fully present and awake.

- Now close your eyes, if that feels comfortable for you.

- Become very aware of what is going on with you right now. What thoughts do you have? As best you can, just note any thoughts as mental events. As you take note of them, see if you can sense any physical feelings associated with them. Do you sense any emotions? If you notice any discomfort or unpleasant feelings, don't try to push them away or shut them out; just acknowledge that they are there. You might say, "Ah, here you are; that's how it is right now." And similarly with sensations in your body, you might say, "Is that a tension? A holding? What does it feel like? Okay, that's how it is right now."

Step 2: Focus on the movements of the breath.

- Focus on your abdomen, the rise and fall of your breath. This minute will be spent focusing on the movement of your abdominal wall, moment by moment, breath by breath, as best as you can. When you feel the breath moving in, you know it is moving in. And when you feel your breath moving out, you know it is moving out. See if you can focus your attention on any patterns of your breath sensations, whether they are at your nostrils, chest, or belly. And use your breath as your anchor.

Step 3: Expand awareness to sensations in entire body.
You might notice tightness or other sensations related to a sense of tension in your shoulders, neck, back, or face. In addition, you might notice sensations of your breath and your body as they emerge, linger, and fade away.

At the end of step 3 you can open your eyes.

Some people choose to do this practice every day. Others use it only before an event that they expect will be stressful. Some women use it before—or even during—sexual activity. In your journal, keep track of where and when you practice it and any observations you make about physical and mental sensations you noticed. Try to provide as much detail as you can.

STRUGGLES AND STRATEGIES

The struggles below relate to both the Mindfulness of Thoughts practice and the Self-Observation and Touch exercise. As always, the strategies to address the struggles are meant as a guide, and I encourage you to come up with your own.

THE STRUGGLE: I CANNOT SEEM TO OBSERVE MY THOUGHTS WITHOUT GETTING CAUGHT UP IN THEM.
In the Mindfulness of Thoughts practice, I introduced you to the analogy of watching your thoughts from a distance, as if you were sitting on the bank of a stream. This is challenging for many people, especially if your thoughts quickly pull you into their content!

Strategies

- Imagine yourself sitting on the bank of the stream and watching your thoughts flow by.

- Or imagine a train going by, with every boxcar representing a different thought. You don't try to hop on board but simply watch it go by as you stand alongside the train track.

- Or imagine that your thoughts are clouds and you are watching them from the ground.

- Limit the time you focus on your thoughts. Try it for one minute, then move your focus to your breath. After a few moments, see if you can shift your focus to your thoughts again. With practice, you may be able to stay with your thoughts for progressively longer periods.

THE STRUGGLE: I FEEL UNCOMFORTABLE TOUCHING MY OWN GENITALS.

As already noted, many women have never explored their own genitals through touch, and the thought of doing so makes them feel uncomfortable or even embarrassed. You might have thoughts come up such as "This is wrong" or "This is inappropriate" or "Someone will walk in and see me."

Strategies

- Read the exercise over a few times and visualize yourself doing it before you actually try it.

- Treat this as a mindful exercise but instead of observing the sensations in your whole body, you are observing, through touch, the sensations in your vulva.

- Be patient. Be kind. Try to observe mindfully and leave judgments aside.

TIME TO PRACTICE

Over the next few days, try the Mindfulness of Thoughts practice as often as possible. You have already practiced the Body Scan and Mindful Movement for a couple of weeks now, and you have likely developed some skill in noticing sensations in your body and your breath. Now you are going to try to notice the frequency, quality, and any emotional tone of your thoughts, but *not* their content. The more you can practice mindfulness of thoughts, the more you will be able to sit beside the river bank without getting swept in, even when the river looks in danger of breaking its banks. Eventually, this will be a skill you can start to integrate into all of your activities, including your sexual ones.

I also invite you to try the informal Focusing practice in this chapter, and to bring awareness to any thoughts you have about your body. Try to embrace awareness and acceptance of whatever thoughts come up in relation to your body.

Try to use the 3-Minute Breathing Space practice at least once a day. Remember to keep track of where and when you are using it to see if any patterns emerge as to where you find this practice the most useful.

Finally, try to do the informal Self-Observation and Touch practice twice before you move on to chapter 5. Try to set aside at least fifteen minutes for it. If you stop or get interrupted, try again another day.

5

When Difficulties Arise during Sex

USING MINDFULNESS TO ADDRESS EMOTIONAL AND PHYSICAL DIFFICULTIES WITH SEX

The science indicates that people with a sexual dysfunction are more likely than others to also have emotional or physical difficulties, or both. Chronic and unresolved trauma or depression can directly affect sexual response and even surface as flashbacks during sexual activity. Chronic pain can lead to lack of interest in sex and problems with sexual desire. Whether the challenge takes an emotional form (memories, thoughts, negative emotions) or physical form (chronic pain, tension, discomfort), it can interfere with sex—before, during, or after sexual activity—by reducing your motivation for sex, distracting you during sex, or interfering with your ability to appreciate the rewarding aspects of sexual activity. Sometimes these forms of suffering can stand in the way of any participation in sexual activity.

This chapter focuses on how mindfulness can help with emotional and physical difficulties by challenging our tendency to ignore such difficulties and instead helping us to face them, which the scientific research tells us is the far more effective approach. We will first consider a mindfulness practice that brings awareness to mental or emotional discomfort. Later in the chapter we will practice a mindfulness exercise that brings awareness to physical discomfort.

FORMAL EXERCISE 5:
WORKING WITH DIFFICULTY MEDITATION

In chapter 4 you practiced observing your thoughts from a distance, as if you were sitting on the bank of a stream, watching them float by. Sometimes intentionally watching thoughts leads to their disappearing.

But what happens if we *intentionally* want to bring up upsetting thoughts? Can you imagine yourself mindfully watching those negative thoughts from a distance without becoming immersed in them? Because we so often have upsetting thoughts in our day-to-day life, including during sexual activity, being able to observe them mindfully while having compassion for ourselves and without reacting is an important skill.

In the following mindfulness practice, I will ask you to bring to mind a difficult situation that provokes a mild level of emotional discomfort for you. Maybe it is the memory of an argument with a family member or coworker. Maybe it is a longstanding stress or worry in your life. Maybe it is the feeling you had after you received some sad news. I suggest you bring up a difficult situation that is low on the scale from being not at all upsetting to being extremely upsetting—perhaps a memory that measures 3 out of 10 in level of distress for you. When you can practice relating to these difficult situations with mindfulness, you will be better equipped to manage them when they arise in real life.

WHAT YOU WILL NEED

· A chair, ideally high-back
· A quiet space (remember that no space will be totally silent, and that is okay!)
· Comfortable socks or shoes
· Your journal

This meditation will take about fifteen minutes.

STEP-BY-STEP GUIDE TO WORKING
WITH DIFFICULTY MEDITATION

- Settle into a comfortable sitting position.

- Make any adjustments to enable you to sit as comfortably as you can with an erect and dignified posture. Check to see that your spine, neck, and head are in alignment. Your feet should be flat on the floor. Let your hands rest on your thighs or in your lap.

- Allow your eyes to gently close if this feels comfortable, or if you prefer, choose a spot in front of you, either straight ahead or downward, and focus on it with a soft gaze.

- Settle into the sensations of sitting, just as you find them, right here, right now. Allow your attention to move fluidly from sensation to sensation, as each arises and fades in prominence.

- Do your best to stay alert and mentally focused throughout the practice.

- When you are ready, move the focus of your attention from the sensations of your body sitting here to focus more narrowly on the sensations of breathing. Become aware of each in-breath and each out-breath as they follow, one after the other.

- Whenever you notice that your attention has moved to a physical sensation elsewhere in your body, a sound, or a thought that is more predominant, momentarily take this to be the new focus of your attention. When this is no longer predominant, bring the focus of your attention back to the sensations of breathing.

- Continue to do this for a few minutes.

- In this practice, it is often helpful to follow your breath in one part of your body. There are a number of places in the body where the breath makes itself known. Focus your attention on the patterns of physical sensations at your nostrils, as your breath moves into and out of your body. As you breathe in, feel the sensations at your nostrils as the cool air is drawn into your body. And then, on the out-breath, feel the sensations of friction or pressure at your nostrils as the warm air leaves your body.

- You do not need to breathe in any particular way or use your breath to get anywhere. Just let your breath move in and out naturally.

- When you are ready, move the focus of attention down your body to your chest and notice sensations in this area. Feel the expansion of your chest as you breathe in and the falling away of your chest as you breathe out. Tune in to this gentle rhythm of the chest's rising and falling as you breathe. Observe the sensations of breathing in this part of your body for a few minutes.

- When you are ready again, move the focus of your attention farther down your body to your abdomen and your belly. Feel the expansion of your belly as it rises on the in-breath and the gentle deflation of your belly on the out-breath. As best as you can, focus all the way through as your breath enters your body on the in-breath, and all the way through as your breath leaves your body on the out-breath. Perhaps notice the slight pauses between one in-breath and the following out-breath, and between one out-breath and the following in-breath.

- Now you may choose to either stay with the breath at your belly or move to another place where your breath makes itself known to you most vividly. Keep your focus there for a minute. You can close your eyes and continue for a few minutes.

- Whenever you notice that you have forgotten about noticing your breath sensations because your attention was engaged in or identifying with the content of a thought, congratulate yourself on becoming aware of that. This is perfectly okay. It's simply what minds do. It doesn't mean you've made a mistake or you're doing something wrong. Notice what your attention was engaged with and then turn your attention back with kindness to the sensations of breathing in the region you are focusing on.

· When you are ready, expand your field of awareness to include your entire body, from the top of your head to the soles of your feet. Pay careful attention to the many individual sensations that arise and pass away within this larger field of awareness, wherever they may be located in your body. Allow your attention to move fluidly from sensation to sensation, wherever they arise in your body, momentarily focusing on each one, as it rises and fades in prominence, and, without straining, observing each as clearly as possible.

· Perhaps notice the sensations where your body makes contact with the floor or the chair. Bring a friendly, interested attention to sensations of touch or pressure, such as sensations in your buttocks where they make contact with the chair or in your hands where they rest on your thighs or on each other. Perhaps notice the sensations of breathing at your nostrils, chest, or belly.

· While you are sitting, if you notice that your attention keeps being pulled away to difficult or painful thoughts or emotions, you can explore something different from what we've been practicing up until now.

· In the exercises you've done up until now, when you have been sitting and notice that your attention has become engaged in the content of a thought or a story, I have asked you to simply notice what your attention has been engaged with and then gently and firmly escort your attention back to your breath or body or back to whatever you intended to be focusing on.

· Now you can explore a different way to respond. Instead of bringing your attention back from an upsetting thought or feeling, allow the thought or feeling to be the focus of your attention.

- Then shift your attention to your body, becoming aware of any physical sensations that arise in your body as you observe the upsetting thought or emotion.

- Then, when you have identified such sensations, deliberately move the focus of your attention to the part of your body where these sensations are strongest. This could be your face, your throat, your chest, your abdomen, or another area. Bring a kind attention to this region, not for the purpose of changing the sensations, but rather to observe them and see them clearly.

- If no difficulties or concerns come up and you want to explore this new approach, I invite you to deliberately bring to mind a current difficulty in your life. It should be something you don't mind staying with for a short while during your practice. It should be approximately a 3 or 4 out of 10 on your distress scale, and it should be a thought, emotion, or memory that you experience as somewhat unpleasant and somewhat unresolved. This might be a misunderstanding or an argument, or a situation where you feel somewhat angry, regretful, or guilty about something that has happened. If nothing comes to mind, you could choose something difficult or upsetting from your past.

- Once you have focused on that difficult situation, take your time to tune in to any physical sensations in your body that the difficulty evokes.

- Observe the feelings that are arising in your body, becoming mindful of the range of physical sensations. Direct your focus of attention to the region of your body where the sensations are strongest and see if you can welcome those difficult sensations as if you were extending your arms to make space for them.

· This gesture of welcome might include gently observing your physical sensations and watching their intensity shift up and down from one moment to the next.

· Whenever a thought, emotion, sound (such as breathing or noises in your stomach), or sensation in another area of your body becomes more prominent than the sensations associated with the difficult memory, take this to be the new focus of your attention until it is no longer predominant. Then bring your attention back to the region of your body you are focusing on.

· Once your attention has settled on the sensations in your body associated with the difficulty and they are vividly present in the field of your awareness, unpleasant as they might be, try to deepen your acceptance of and openness to whatever sensations are there by saying to yourself from time to time, "It is here now. It is okay to be open to it. Whatever it is, it's already here. Let me be open to it."

· As you soften your attitude toward those difficult thoughts and emotions, and their physical sensations in your body, and as you open to them even more, you might say to yourself, "Softening" or "Opening" on each out-breath.

· Softening. Opening.

· Remain focused on the sensations in your body, observing them and your relationship to them as they arise. Breathe along with those sensations and with the upsetting thought or memory. Let the sensations be just as they are. Accept them as they are.

· Remember that by saying to yourself, "It's already here" or "It's okay," you are not judging the original situation or saying that everything is fine; rather, you are simply guiding your awareness and attention to those thoughts or memories and remaining open to them.

- Observing difficult thoughts, emotions, and sensations as they are and accepting them as they are does not mean you are giving in to them.

- You do not have to like these feelings. In fact, it is natural not to want to have them around. You may find it helpful to say to yourself, "It's okay not to want these feelings, but they're already here, so let me be open to them."

- If you choose, you can also experiment with expanding the focus of your attention around the sensations to include the sensations of breathing. Allow your attention to focus on the body sensation or breath sensation that is most prominent moment to moment, as each arises, lingers, and fades away.

- When you notice that the sensations in your body are no longer pulling on your attention to the same degree, simply focus your attention on the sensations of breathing.

- Spend the next few minutes in open awareness of anywhere in your body that the difficult thoughts or emotions take you. As you move your attention there, continue to be open to these thoughts or emotions, accepting them just as they are. Let go of the need to change them or turn them off.

- As we move into the last few moments of this meditation, I invite you to return to your sensations of breathing. Become aware of each in-breath and each out-breath as they follow, one after another.

- When you're ready, allow your eyes to open if they were closed. If your eyes were open, raise them to look straight ahead of you now. Shift your focus from sensations in your body to the words on the page as you further consider your experience.

- Finally, take a few deep breaths before you move on to the Inquiry.

THE INQUIRY

Read the Inquiry questions silently to yourself while you remain present in your body and breath sensations. After you have read each one that relates to question 1, you can spend time reflecting on the answer, or you can write your answers down in your journal. Then do the same with questions 2 and 3.

QUESTION 1. What did you notice during this practice as you evoked a difficult memory or situation?

Could you conjure up a difficult situation that was about a 3 or 4 out of 10 in intensity? If you feel comfortable, write down what the difficult memory was that you conjured up.

What sensations came up for you during this practice as you held that difficult situation at the center of your attention? Can you describe those sensations in more detail? Did they change over time? If they changed, what changes did you notice? For example, did you notice sensations more strongly in particular parts of your body?

Did you notice particular thoughts, or mental sensations? Could you observe those mental sensations from a distance, as if you were sitting on the bank of a stream? Did those mental sensations change in intensity as you continued to pay attention? If so, in what way?

Did the difficult memory evoke any emotions? If so, did those emotions show up in your body somewhere? And if they did, could you remain focused there?

What was it like to bring an open acceptance to the sensations that came up as you evoked this difficult memory? What did it feel like to be open to them with compassion? How did you know you were reacting with compassion and acceptance toward the difficulty you evoked?

Take your time in answering these questions. They are challenging.

QUESTION 2. How was tuning in to difficult thoughts, emotions, and physical sensations in this way different from how you might usually relate to difficulties?

In this practice you deliberately brought to mind a difficult situation. When you have an upsetting thought or image or feeling in your day-to-day life, what do you typically do? Was the way you brought attention to it now new for you? I also invited you to open your arms to whatever feelings arose as a result, whether they were positive, negative, or neutral. If that was also new for you, what did that feel like? Try to be as detailed as possible about how this experience of moving toward a difficulty resembled or differed from how you typically experience difficult memories or emotions. In what ways was it similar? In what ways was it different? Take your time as you write your answers down in your journal.

QUESTION 3. How was this practice of mindfulness of a difficulty relevant to your sexuality?

How was staying with emotional discomfort in this soft, open, accepting, and compassionate way relevant to your sexual desire or sexual arousal? You practiced staying with physical tension and discomforts during the mindful stretching practice earlier in this book, but this time you were staying with an emotional discomfort. How might this way of "being with" emotional discomfort be relevant to your sexual health? Were you surprised by your degree or intensity of self-compassion, and if so, could your ability to be compassionate to yourself be helpful when you encounter sexual difficulties? Did you experience physical sensations in your body during the emotional upset in an open and nonjudgmental way, observing all of the physical sensations just as they are? If so, how might that experience benefit your sexual health? Don't worry about trying to find the "right" answer—there are none! This is an opportunity for you to contemplate how extending this kind of acceptance to difficulty could be useful to you sexually and personally.

END OF THE WORKING WITH DIFFICULTY MEDITATION

Take a moment to stand, stretch, and maybe look outside. Remember to congratulate yourself for completing this practice. This was not the first mindfulness practice that involved paying attention to a difficulty. In the Mindful Movement practice in chapter 3, you brought compassionate awareness to physical tensions in your body. Remember how long you held some of those poses? This Working with Difficulty meditation also involved taking a compassionate approach to difficulties, but this time it was an emotional one.

Perhaps you found this practice difficult. If so, you are not alone. Here are some of the comments women in our mindful sex groups have made after doing the Working with Difficulty meditation:

- I can honestly say that I have never "opened myself compassionately" to upsetting memories. This was a first for me.

- Usually when I am reminded of an argument, I try to bury it by distracting myself with something else because thinking about the argument is just too upsetting for me. It was quite different for me to not distract myself.

- If I am thinking about a conflict going on in my life right now, I can't seem to shake it. I imagine the words the other person said to me over and over again. I re-imagine it in my mind as if it were being played out in real life. In this practice, I really tried to just watch what I was thinking and feeling while imagining myself sitting at the side of the river. I had truly never tried that before.

· I noticed that even though I was bringing up an upsetting memory in my mind, there were lots of physical sensations in my body that became more intense the more I brought up the difficulty. I had no idea just how much thoughts or feelings could trigger physical sensations in my body!

· When you asked me to cultivate compassion toward my upsetting thoughts, I imagined myself as a child with open arms and a smile looking at my emotions. It actually helped to smile at them, as it neutralized their intensity a bit.

In the mindful sex groups, many of the women have said that they found this practice of bringing mindfulness to a difficulty to be quite relevant to their own sexual lives. I always ask them how it might be useful for helping them to navigate their sexual concerns. Here are some of their responses:

· I often worry during sex, and the worry leads to a cascade of sensations in my body, sweaty palms, thoughts about disappointing my partner, and then the cycle continues. The mindfulness of a difficulty has been allowing me to turn toward those emotions, thoughts, and physical sensations, rather than away from them. When I do this during sexual activity, I notice that they are less scary. Less intense. And with more focus, they eventually fade so that I can return my attention to the much more pleasurable sensations of sex!

· Sometimes during sex I will have a vivid memory of my experience with sexual violence. It sounds awful, but I can sometimes elicit a memory so vivid of this assault that it feels as if it was happening in real time. Obviously this blocks the sex I am having with my partner. By practicing working through an emotional difficulty in my mindfulness practice, it has given me the confidence that if such upsetting thoughts come up during sex, I can try to let them be without reacting to them, and that is probably a far healthier way of experiencing those memories than what I had been doing.

- I feel so guilty about my lack of interest in sex that when my partner and I engage in sex, it starts to feel good, but then I might have a memory of times in the past when it did not go well, and that memory leads me to literally turn off my arousal. This practice of being mindful of upsetting memories and tuning in to my body sensations during it will be something I definitely try in the future when negative thoughts come up. I think it could be a great way to help me manage the guilt I feel.

USING MINDFULNESS TO WORK THROUGH AN EMOTIONAL DIFFICULTY CAN IMPROVE ASPECTS OF SEXUALITY

Are you prone to having negative thoughts during sexual activity? Perhaps sex leads you to feel guilty, bad about yourself, angry, or another strong emotion? We know that women who experience low desire, difficulties with arousal, painful sex, or lack of pleasure in sex might be especially prone to having negative thoughts and strong, negative emotions about and during sex. Perhaps they start out feeling positive, but then their minds drift toward negative feelings and thoughts. Mindfulness can help to soften the intensity of these negative feelings and allow these women to refocus on more sensual and pleasurable ones.

If you have experienced abusive or nonconsensual sex in the past, your emotional memory will be much stronger than the one you elicited in the meditation. For some women, sexual arousal when they are having sex can be the trigger for unpleasant memories of traumatic sexual experiences. Although the current research cannot tell us just how common this is, in my research program we have encountered many women who have told us that consensual sexual activity with a partner can trigger flashbacks to past sexual abuse. For some women, the traumatic memories are so vivid and upsetting that they avoid sex with their current partner altogether.

If you are having repeated and intrusive memories of sexual abuse, think about seeking help from a qualified mental health practitioner to guide you through the steps of confronting and working through those negative feelings and memories. For some women, memories of abuse remain buried and never affect their sex lives. For others, there can be a decades-long struggle with feelings of fear, guilt, shame, and anxiety after an episode or episodes of abuse. If you have an unresolved trauma related to any history of unwanted or upsetting occurrences from your past, think about seeking psychological help from a professional, as it could be directly affecting your sexual well-being today.

MINDFULNESS OF PAIN

Up to 40 percent of people in the general population live with chronic pain. Many more than that live with intermittent and less severe but still upsetting pain, discomfort, and various ailments. Remember the sexual response cycle you learned about in chapter 3? You learned how information from the body, the mind, and memories is processed in the brain to produce sexual arousal. Pain can block this information from being processed and prevent you from experiencing sexual arousal and responsive sexual desire.

If you are in pain, your motivation to participate in activities that can intensify that pain, such as sex, is likely to wane. Research shows, however, that repeated mindfulness practice can help lessen the intensity of pain and reduce the amount of emotional suffering you feel when you are living with chronic pain. It turns "When will this pain go away so I can start living?" into "I will live alongside this pain."

FORMAL EXERCISE 6:
PROVOKING A MILD PAIN MEDITATION

In this practice, I invite you to turn your attention toward an area of discomfort (or pain or tension) in your body. You will not be dwelling on the discomfort or the source of the discomfort. Instead, you will use the attention skills you used to tune in to physical sensations in your body in the practices earlier in this workbook to move even closer to the bare sensations that make up the area of pain or discomfort. And as with the Working with Difficulty meditation you practiced earlier, I will invite you to focus on an area of discomfort that is relatively low on the pain intensity meter—probably something about a 3 or 4 out of 10 in pain intensity. Ready?

WHAT YOU WILL NEED

- A chair, ideally high-back
- A quiet space (remember that no space will be totally silent, and that is okay!)
- Comfortable socks or shoes
- Your journal

This practice will take about twenty minutes.

STEP-BY-STEP GUIDE TO PROVOKING A MILD PAIN MEDITATION

- Start by settling into a comfortable sitting position. Take the time now to make any adjustments to enable you to sit as comfortably as you can in an upright and dignified posture. Check that your spine, neck, and head are in alignment and your feet are flat on the floor. Let your hands rest on your thighs or in your lap. Allow your eyes to gently close if this feels comfortable, or if you prefer, you can choose a spot in front of you and focus on it with a soft gaze.

- Settle into the sensations of sitting, just as you find them, right here, right now. Allow your attention to move easily from sensation to sensation, as each arises and fades in prominence.

- Do your best to stay alert and mentally focused throughout the practice.

- When you are ready, move your focus of attention from the sensations of your body sitting here to focus more narrowly on the sensations of breathing. Become aware of each in-breath and each out-breath, one after the other.

- Whenever you notice that your attention has moved to a physical sensation elsewhere in your body, a sound, or a thought that is more predominant, take this to be your new focus for attention for a moment. When it is no longer predominant, bring the focus of your attention back to the sensations of breathing.

- Take a moment to notice where in your body your breath is making itself known. Turn your attention now to the patterns of physical sensations first at the nostrils, as your breath moves into and out of your body. As you breathe in, feel the sensations at your nostrils as the cooler air is drawn into your body. And then, on the out-breath, feel the sensations of friction or pressure at your nostrils as the warm air leaves your body. You don't need to breathe in any particular way or use your breath to get anywhere. Just let your breath be there as it is.

- When you are ready, move the focus of your attention down your body to your chest and notice sensations in this area. Feel the expansion of your chest as you breathe in and the falling away of your chest as you breathe out. Tune in to this gentle rhythm of your chest's rising and falling as you breathe. Observe the sensations of breathing in this part of your body.

- When you are ready again, move the focus of your attention farther down your body to your abdomen and belly. Feel the expansion of your belly as it rises on the in-breath and the gentle deflation of the belly on the out-breath. As best as you can, focus as closely as possible while your breath enters your body on the in-breath, and all the way through as the breath leaves your body on the out-breath. Perhaps notice the slight pauses between one in-breath and the following out-breath, and between one out-breath and the following in-breath.

· You might choose now to stay with the breath at your belly or to move to another place where the breath makes itself known to you and stay with that as the primary focus of your attention.

· Now I am going to ask you to evoke a mild unpleasant physical sensation by holding one of your arms up over your head (with or without the support of your other arm) for the duration of this exercise.

· Go ahead and lift your arm up now. Hold it for a little while and breathe through it and into it.

· Bring your attention to the individual smaller sensations that make up the increasingly intense sensations in your arm. For example, are the smaller sensations sharp or dull? Does the intensity of the sensations change over time? Can you notice the very beginning and end of each of the smaller sensations that make up the larger experience of intensity?

· See if you can define the physical boundary of the sensations— how far they extend—and what characteristics the intense sensations are made up of.

· Continue to keep your arm in the air.

· While you are observing these characteristics, see if you can notice how your attention tends to want to move away from any uncomfortable sensations. This resistance to simply allowing the uncomfortable sensations to exist and be with them in the moment is an example of aversion. It can be quite useful to get to know the signs of such resistance arising in order to be able to recognize it more easily. If you can, focus on the resistance to the uncomfortable sensations. Do not attempt to remove the resistance. Simply pay careful attention to it.

- If the resistance disappears, bring your attention back to the physical sensations that make up the unpleasant sensations in your arm.

- When the resistance arises again, pay careful attention to it in the moment. Keep returning to the physical qualities of the intense sensations and then noticing the aversion to the intense sensations when it occurs. Notice also if the feelings of resistance trigger any additional physical sensations, such as muscular tension, straining, a slight furrowing of the brow, sensations of sleepiness, sensations of restlessness, or subtle manipulations of the breath, as well as follow-on emotions, such as fear, or wanting to do something to make the uncomfortable sensation go away.

- Try to notice all the physical and mental sensations of wanting the discomfort in your arm to go away and breathe through it. Notice any disliking. Notice that aversion is impermanent—just like any other sensation.

- You may now lower your raised arm. Rest in stillness for a minute.

- Observe the changes in sensations that come with returning your arm to your side or to your lap. See if you can also note any changes in the sensations that arise from the movement of your arm.

- Notice if there are any mental sensations now. Continue to breathe through them.

- Next, try to find a location in your body where there is a pleasant physical sensation and pay careful attention to it. Maybe it is an area of pleasant warmth or comfort. Maybe it is an area that is free of any discomfort. Move your attention there now.

- See if you can notice all the various physical sensations that make up that pleasant feeling or sensations of comfort. Observe these sensations in as much detail as possible. See if you can notice whether your attention is trying to cling to those pleasant sensations. Notice if there is a desire for the pleasant sensations to continue or increase in intensity and how your attention might be very focused on those feelings, rather than simply allowing the pleasant sensation to exist as it is and just rest with it in the moment, without a strong need to cling to it.

- The desire to remain with pleasant feelings is an example of attachment to bare sensations.

- It is very useful to learn to spot the signs of attachment so that you can recognize it more easily. If you can, focus on the attachment to the pleasant sensation. Do not attempt to remove the attachment. Simply pay careful attention to it.

- When the attachment disappears, bring your attention back to the physical sensations that make up the area of comfort or pleasant feeling. When attachment arises again, pay careful attention to it.

- Keep returning to the pleasant physical sensations and then switching to noticing the attachment to the pleasant sensations when it occurs. Notice also if there are any follow-on physical sensations associated with the attachment, such as muscular tension, straining, changes in the breath, or a slight leaning forward, or follow-on thoughts such as fear that the pleasant sensations will go away, wanting to do something to make the pleasant sensations stay or increase in intensity, or wanting to look for other pleasant sensations in your body.

- Try to notice all the physical and mental sensations of wanting the transient pleasant physical sensation to linger. Notice if there is any liking.

- Notice that attachment is impermanent—just like any other sensation.

- Continue to observe in this way for a few more moments.

- As you come to the end of this practice, form the intention to bring this moment-to-moment noticing of sensations with you as you continue to reflect on your experience.

- You may want to wiggle your toes and fingers, noticing sensations of movement. You may wish to congratulate yourself on having taken the time and expended the energy to nourish yourself in this way, and to remember that this state of awareness is accessible to you by simply paying attention to sensations, such as those of the in-breath and the out-breath, in any moment, no matter what is happening, at any time of the day.

THE INQUIRY

As you read through the following three questions, consider writing your answers down in your journal. You might also compare your answers to these questions about mindfulness toward a physical difficulty with the answers you provided about mindfulness toward an emotional difficulty.

QUESTION 1. What did you notice during this practice when you were invited to pay attention to sensations in your arm after holding it up for a while?

When you first held up your arm, you may have just noticed the physical movement as you moved it from its starting position to its end position. However, gravity makes its presence known fairly quickly, and you probably soon needed to exert muscular tension to keep your arm up. Even without holding anything in your hand, the weight of your arm can elicit intense sensations.

Even pain. Did you notice a desire to put your arm down? Where did you notice that? And what did you do? What kinds of mental sensations came up as you held your arm above your head? Did they change the longer you held your arm up?

Did you notice an aversion to the sensations—for example, maybe wanting to distract yourself from the increasingly intense sensations in your arm? Where did aversion show up for you?

Take your time in answering these questions. They are challenging.

QUESTION 2. How was tuning in to intense physical sensations in this way different from how you might usually relate to similar intense physical sensations or pain in your body?

In this practice you deliberately tuned in to pain. I encouraged you to focus on its physical qualities instead of labeling it as pain. In fact, I did not use the term "pain" at all during this practice. How was tuning in to the physical intensity different from how you normally pay attention to physical discomforts? Are you quick to shift position to lessen pain? Perhaps you rub the area that feels uncomfortable or look for other signs of triggers that are making the pain worse. Here I asked you just to notice the intensity with curiosity and kindness. What difference did taking that approach make for you?

Take your time as you write your answers down in your journal.

QUESTION 3. How was this practice of bringing mindfulness toward an area of physical intensity in your body relevant to your sexuality?

Consider how bringing mindful awareness to a physical discomfort could be useful to you during sexual activity. Do you ever experience pain or tension in your body during sex that seems to dominate your attention? Did you learn something about relating to discomfort in a compassionate way during this practice that you could imagine applying to your sexual encounters when you experience discomfort?

How was staying with physical discomfort in this way, being open to it with compassion and without labeling it as pain, relevant to your sexual desire or sexual arousal? If you experience pain or discomfort during sexual activity, what do you usually do? Was there anything that surprised you in this practice that you might consider applying to your sexual experiences should you ever feel physical tension or pain?

The first formal exercise in this chapter had you practice bringing awareness to an emotional difficulty; in this practice you brought awareness to a physical difficulty. In both cases, you brought mindfulness and compassionate self-awareness to something difficult, and perhaps something you might typically avoid. Can you apply anything you learned from these two practices to your sexual experiences? If so, write about this in your journal.

END OF THE PROVOKING A MILD PAIN MEDITATION
Congratulations on finishing this Provoking a Mild Pain meditation plus the guided Inquiry. You might wish to stand and move around before continuing.

HOW MIGHT MINDFULNESS OF PAIN IMPROVE ASPECTS OF YOUR SEXUALITY?

If you experience chronic pain, you have likely tried multiple treatments to reduce its intensity or persistence. If those treatments have not alleviated your pain, you might have asked yourself, "Why me?" soon followed by "Will this pain ever end?" and "Why don't my doctors know how to make me feel better?" Before you know it, you're asking yourself, "Will this pain get worse and interfere with my day-to-day activities? Will I have to quit my job? Will my partner leave me out of frustration? Am I destined to be alone living with chronic pain?" You can see how quickly one thought ("Why me?") leads to the next and then the next and then the next. Do you see the stream passing by, filled with more and more thoughts? Perhaps you have jumped into the stream and are being swept downstream in the multitude of thoughts about your pain. Neuroscientific research examining the brain during pain episodes indicates that progressively negative thoughts and emotions about pain can make the pain feel more intense. In other words, focusing on your suffering can make you suffer more.

The mindfulness meditation you just completed is similar to many of the practices in the earlier chapters in which you practiced following your breath and then bringing more intense sensations into the foreground and observing their characteristics—burning, tightness, irritation, soreness, and tension—and then trying to experience those sensations very clearly, just as they were, without judgment or interpretation. By noticing that the sensations change from moment to moment, you might observe that what you would typically label as "pain" is actually a series of momentary physical sensations that occur in quick succession, one after another.

As you move through this meditation, you become aware of the mental sensations that are associated with the physical intensity and label them. They might be feelings of anger, fear, worry, despair, or hopelessness. Over time, if you continue with your mindfulness practice, you might be able to observe the cause-and-effect relationship between the sensations of pain, the mental reactions to those sensations, the increase in physical tension as a result of those reactions, and possibly the increase in intensity of the physical sensations of pain as a result.

You might also observe that simply noticing the mental sensations, with kindness and compassion toward yourself, can stop the cycle and might reduce the intensity of the pain sensations. And you might observe that your aversion to those sensations was a source of your suffering.

Mindfully noticing sensations of intensity—what we would normally call pain—with compassion and acceptance can significantly reduce suffering and in turn reduce the intensity of your pain. Tuning in to those areas of discomfort lessens how much interference they cause and how much pain they provoke. My research team and our sexual medicine clinician colleagues at the University of British Columbia have assessed the value of group mindfulness for women with a chronic genital, or vulvo-vaginal, pain condition called Provoked Vestibulodynia (you may recall that I mentioned this condition in chapter 1). After eight weeks of practice in a group, all the participants experienced dramatic decreases in their vulvo-vaginal pain. Their pain continued to decrease during the six months after the mindfulness group ended. And when we followed up at the one–year point after their mindfulness sessions were complete, we discovered it had decreased even more. The participants were therefore motivated to continue to practice mindfulness because of the tangible benefits they experienced—not only in terms of their vulvo-vaginal pain but also in how much they focused on the pain and how much they catastrophized about it.

The two mindfulness exercises you have just practiced—Working with Difficulty (in which you practiced mindfulness of an emotional pain) and Provoking a Mild Pain (in which you practiced mindfulness of a physical pain)—are relevant to your sexuality. By observing patterns in your mind and perhaps its tendency to push away negative feelings and cling to positive feelings, you might be able to recognize when these patterns emerge during sexual activity—perhaps when pleasure and arousal arise and you find yourself clinging to those sensations, or when vulvo-vaginal pain arises and you find yourself avoiding those feelings. What do you think? Can you imagine applying this new way of relating to discomfort in your own sex life? If so, how? Write down your thoughts about how you might do this in your journal.

STRUGGLES AND STRATEGIES

The struggles covered below pertain to both the Working with Difficulty meditation and the Provoking a Mild Pain meditation. If the strategies listed below do not resonate with you, record your own strategy in your journal.

THE STRUGGLE: ALL OF MY EMOTIONAL DIFFICULTIES ARE VERY UPSETTING AND I DO NOT HAVE ANY THAT ARE MILD. In the Working with Difficulty meditation, I suggested that you pull up a memory of a past (resolved) issue or recall a current one that is relatively low on the scale from 0 (not emotionally upsetting at all) to 10 (extremely emotionally upsetting). That is because it is more challenging to apply the mindfulness skills of observing nonjudgmentally when the difficulty you are recalling is quite upsetting or evokes a high level of intense emotions for you.

Strategies

- Consider recalling a past emotional conflict that has already been resolved.

- Consider inventing a conflict in your imagination that is of low intensity and relates to something that might happen in your life.

- Consider bringing up an emotional conflict that someone you care about has experienced.

THE STRUGGLE: I FIND IT CHALLENGING TO NOT LABEL PAIN AS PAIN DURING THE PROVOKING A MILD PAIN MEDITATION. AFTER ALL, IT IS PAINFUL!

In the Provoking a Mild Pain meditation, I encouraged you to tune in to the bare sensations of pain without labeling them as pain. The word "pain" is emotionally laden. It conjures up memories, stories, and feelings. I would like you to feel sensations in your body without them automatically triggering story lines of their own.

Strategies

· You might write some guiding questions in your journal to take note of when you are eliciting the physical tension: Where do you feel it? What does it feel like? Does it radiate or remain fixed? What level of intensity is it? Does the intensity change?

· Imagine describing those feelings to someone who has never experienced pain. If you are not relying on pain to describe a sensation, you must rely on the physical attributes of the sensation to describe it.

TIME TO PRACTICE

Over the next week, try both of these new mindfulness practices, beginning with the Working with Difficulty meditation. Again, choose a situation that is likely to cause a relatively low level of emotional upset. Use your journal to track the date of your practice, and any physical and mental sensations you became aware of during the practice.

When you try the Provoking a Mild Pain meditation you can follow the step-by-step guide to eliciting a new pain by holding up your arm for an extended period of time. If, however, you are experiencing some kind of chronic pain—such as back pain or a mild headache—you could make that the focus of your practice.

Some participants in our groups have elected to use a dildo or dilator or their own finger at the opening of the vagina to elicit a small amount of vulvo-vaginal pain. The source and location of the pain are not especially important at this point. The most important thing is how you relate to those sensations and how you perceive them. Can you tune in to their bare qualities without getting swept into their story? Again, in your journal, note the date and time of your practice and what physical and mental sensations you observed.

I also encourage you to repeat the informal Self-Observation and Touch practice from chapter 4. If any negative feelings or thoughts or pain arise as you are looking at and touching your body, see if you can apply the skills we have just practiced to dealing with them.

6

Bringing Mindfulness to Sex

PAYING ATTENTION TO SEXUAL SENSATIONS

If you have been working through this workbook at approximately one chapter per week, by now you have spent approximately five weeks integrating a regular mindfulness practice into your life. You have used food, your body sensations, your breath, movement, sounds, and thoughts as the focus for your nonjudgmental awareness practices. You have also practiced tuning in to difficulties—first by deliberately bringing up a painful memory, next by eliciting a mild physical pain, and then by using mindfulness to observe sensations in your body in both scenarios. What have been your most notable observations since you began working through this workbook? Has anything surprised you?

You have also spent time getting to know yourself better by observing your own genitals. Then you added touch as a way of truly knowing the sensations in this area of your body without the expectations that typically accompany sexual activity. Each of the mindfulness and genital awareness exercises have been progressively building on one another to bring us to the point where we will begin to pay attention specifically to sexual sensations.

In this chapter we will more explicitly apply mindfulness to sexual activity. First we will consider how you might begin to bring nonjudgmental present-moment awareness into the sexual activities you are already engaging in. After that, I will give you a mindfulness exercise that you will pair with an erotic tool (another term for erotica, fantasy, and vibrator!).

STAYING PRESENT DURING SEXUAL ACTIVITY

It is normal for a person's attention to move spontaneously to different sensations and thoughts, no matter what type of activity they are participating in. You may have been drawn to this workbook because you were concerned about your mind wandering during sexual activities. Many women with a history of sexual difficulties, and many women without such a history, report that they are often distracted during sexual activity, especially with a partner. Typical distracting thoughts might include: "Will I become aroused?" "Is my partner focusing on me?" "Why is it taking so long to reach orgasm?" They might also include a host of non-sex-related thoughts—everything from "I need to show up on time for work tomorrow" to "Did I remember to turn the oven off?"

Whether these distractions are related to sex or not, they interfere with the sexual response cycle. Mindfulness is the antidote to mind wandering and allows you to refocus on emerging sensations as you receive sexual stimulation. With practice, you can train yourself to more quickly notice when your mind has wandered, redirect your attention back to the present moment, and reconnect with bodily sensations during sex.

Before getting into the specifics of the "how," I want to talk about the "when." Sex does not start at the moment of physical touch or stimulation. I often say to my clients that sex begins the moment your last sexual encounter ends. After a given sexual experience (keep in mind that I define this very broadly as any activity with a partner or alone that leads to sexual pleasure), try to linger in the feelings that emerged, both physically and psychologically. Name the sensations you feel and see if you can remain aware of them for several minutes.

In the days, weeks, and perhaps months after a sexual encounter, take a moment to pause and observe when you feel even mild twinges of sexual excitement. When you sense that you are the object of someone's sexual desire (and ideally that someone is also someone you desire or are attracted to), pay attention to what exactly that feels like. Research indicates that simply sensing that you are the object of another person's sexual desire can be a trigger for your own sexual desire. If you are not paying attention to those sensations, however, they will pass you by. If you are anticipating a sexual encounter, bring up an image of it in your mind and then tune in to your body. Close your eyes so that you can focus on what physical and emotional feelings are there. If you ever find yourself having spontaneous erotic thoughts, and you are in a safe and appropriate situation, let your mind float to a fantasy based on those thoughts and tune in to your body as your mind visualizes the sex that might happen in the coming days or weeks or months.

Now imagine that you are in a situation involving a sexual encounter with a partner. Drawing on the mindfulness skills you have practiced so far, start to deliberately notice sensations more during sexual activity. Whenever you notice that your mind has wandered, start by being kind to yourself. Say, "This is common and it is okay. I can guide my mind back." Responding compassionately to yourself from the outset is important for disrupting the typical self-judgments that come up during sex, especially if you have struggled with your own sexual desire or response in the past. You may be inundated with self-judgment about your sexuality.

When you "drop into the body" at the outset of a sexual encounter, you might find it helpful to first anchor your awareness in a sense of your body as whole, including your posture and the positioning of your body. Take note of the sensations on your face and your facial expression. Then allow your attention to rest on whatever sensation is most prominent, moment to moment. Let's look at some of the specific targets you might focus on.

VISUAL SENSATIONS

· Notice colors, blends, shades, shapes, and movement.

· Periodically look into your partner's eyes. Try to observe their color, shape, and movement.

· Look at your partner's skin. Try to observe tiny details.

· Gaze down at your own body. Rather than "thinking" about your body, observe the bare sensations of your body. Try to take notice of visual aspects you usually do not pay attention to, such as the color of your arms or the length of your torso.

What might be some other visual points to focus your attention on? Write them down in your journal.

TOUCH SENSATIONS

· Notice sensations of temperature, pressure, texture, tingling, roughness, smoothness, hardness, softness, wetness, dryness.

· Bring your attention to the points of contact between your body and your partner's body. Try to stay in one area for a few moments and then move to another point of contact between the two of you.

· Spend time focusing on your own hands and fingertips and the parts of your partner's body that they are touching.

- You can also bring awareness to those places where your body makes contact with the bed or against sheets, blankets, and clothing.

  What might be some other touch points to focus your attention on? Write them down in your journal.

SENSATIONS OF MOVEMENT

- Notice breath sensations in your chest and belly.

- Tune in to the fine details of expanding breath and contracting breath.

- Notice your breath in those places where you are making voluntary movements during sexual activity, such as at your mouth, hands, arms, and legs.

- Scan out from your breath to your body as a whole and tune in to the movements of your body, whether they are single movements or more rhythmic movements.

- Notice also if any movements of your body are in sync with your partner's movements.

  What might be some other sensations of movement to focus your attention on? Write them down in your journal.

QUALITIES OF SOUND

- Listen to the sounds of your breath and your partner's breath. Notice the qualities of the sounds, such as intensity, speed, and pitch.

- Making sounds during sexual activity is normal. What sounds can you tune in to? Rather than identifying or labeling the sound, can you pay attention to its qualities?

- As your bodies come into contact, there may be sounds. Bring your awareness there to see if you can detect specific aspects of the qualities of the sound.

- Sounds often become more pronounced as sexual arousal intensifies and orgasm approaches. Do you sense any intensifying qualities of the sound?

  What might be some other qualities of the sound to focus your attention on? Write them down in your journal.

QUALITIES OF SMELL

- If a candle is burning or an essential oil diffuser is on, can you tune in to the qualities of smell?

- The secretions associated with sexual activity have their own unique smells. How would you describe the qualities of the smells?

- Sometimes smells are pleasing and other times they are not. Can you allow all smells to come to your nose while setting judgment aside and just take note of their qualities? For example, intense or subtle, pungent or sweet.

  What might be some other qualities of smell to focus your attention on? Write them down in your journal.

BRINGING MINDFULNESS TO SENSATIONS CAN ANCHOR YOU IN THE MOMENT

Bringing mindfulness to the sensations of sight, touch, movement, sound, and smell can be an effective way of anchoring you in the moment during sexual activity and preventing you from becoming distracted. By remaining aware of bodily sensations in this way, you can decide whether what you are doing is pleasant to you. If you do find it pleasant, you can continue doing what you're doing; if you do not find it pleasant, perhaps you can adjust what you are doing and how you are doing it.

Which of the different methods of bringing mindfulness into the here-and-now do you think you might use to be present during sexual activity? Write them down in your journal.

WHEN MUSCLE TENSION HINDERS INSTEAD OF HELPS

Many women with a history of sexual difficulties understandably experience anxiety during sexual activity. This anxiety is associated with physiological responses that can make it difficult to become sexually aroused and have comfortable vaginal penetration. Two of the ways in which the body responds to anxiety are to redirect blood flow to the skeletal muscles rather than to the genitals and to produce an increase in muscle tension throughout the body—both of which have an impact on sexual activity.

The pelvic floor is a set of muscles that extend from the front of the pelvis to the very back and that support your organs to keep them in place. If you are anticipating that sex will hurt, your pelvic floor muscles might involuntarily tighten. When that happens, vaginal penetration becomes very difficult—partners often report feeling like they are "hitting a wall" in this situation—which increases the chances of pain and thus reinforces your original belief that sex is going to hurt. This can happen with intercourse, or via penetration with a finger or dildo, a speculum during a pap smear, and even a tampon.

You might find it helpful to periodically quickly scan your body during sexual activity to pick up any sensations of tightness (e.g., in your face, hands, chest, inner thighs, or pelvic floor muscles) or check to see if you are bracing yourself (e.g., clenching your fists and shoulders to get ready for pain). Once you are aware of sensations of tightness in the pelvic floor, you can gently direct your attention to that area and consciously relax the muscles there. If you find that your anxiety or fear is just too intense, you could consider slowing down or postponing sexual activity until you are more relaxed.

SEXUAL SENSATIONS AWARENESS: PAIRING MINDFULNESS WITH EROTIC TOOLS

In our Body Scan and breath awareness practices so far, we have focused on the sensations of the body just as they are. You were not asked to intentionally tense or relax the body or to create sensations. Rather, you brought curiosity and your ability to observe sensations to feelings in your body just as they were. Now I will introduce something a little different.

Before doing the next mindfulness practice, you will first elicit sexual arousal. The idea is that by creating sexual sensations in your body first, your mindfulness practice will then focus on these supercharged, or enhanced, sensations. It is a way to practice mindful sex in a controlled and private situation where you can experiment with noticing stronger sexual sensations and moving your attention to softer and neutral ones.

In our research, we evaluated this exercise on its own (separate from an entire eight-week mindfulness program). Half the participants took part in a mental imagery task in which they vividly imagined themselves taking a walk through a beautiful forest. The other half were guided to take part in a brief Body Scan in which they paid attention to physical sensations. Before doing either the visualization task or the mindfulness exercise, all the participants watched an erotic film while they had their physiological sexual response measured with a vaginal probe. After the film, they completed a questionnaire that asked about their subjective sexual arousal while watching the film. After the visualization or mindfulness exercise, they watched a different erotic film. During the second film, the participants' sexual responses were measured again to see whether the visualization or mindfulness exercise had had any effect on them. Those in the mindfulness group had significantly greater mental sexual arousal than those in the visualization group. In addition, they showed more concordance, or agreement, between their mental sexual arousal and their physiological sexual arousal. In other words, pairing the erotic stimulus with mindfulness led to greater mind-body synchrony around sexual arousal than pairing it with a visualization task.

With that in mind, let's consider three sexual tools that can be used to boost sexual response.

FANTASY: USING YOUR IMAGINATION TO ELICIT SEXUAL AROUSAL

While we can't control the dreams we have at night, we do have a great deal of control over our daydreams and fantasies. That means that you can use fantasy to create, or recreate, your very own sexual scenes to help you when your body is becoming sexually aroused but your mind is distracted and focusing on nonsexual things. Sexual fantasy is a common, natural activity and a way to re-experience pleasurable or exciting situations, behaviors, and events in your mind. It is a way to express your creativity in whatever way you wish. And the best part is that no one needs to know what you are fantasizing about—or even that you are fantasizing.

Fantasy can also help you focus on your body and its sensations. Women often talk about a disconnect between what their body is doing and where their mind is. Concerns about pain, body image, or your partner, for example, can interfere with the natural pleasure you might derive from sexual touch and pull your attention away from the experience, resulting in a disconnect between mind and body. Using fantasy is one way to reconnect your mind and body sexually.

Some women in our mindfulness groups over the years have admitted that they hesitate to fantasize about another person besides their partner. Some worry that thinking about something is as bad as doing it. They feel guilty not only about having a sexual fantasy that involves activities they would never engage in in real life but also about finding such fantasies very arousing. They might feel conflicted and even ashamed. But fantasy is a natural, healthy expression of sexuality, and many women use it to good effect. Research indicates that the types of fantasies women have might have no bearing at all on their sexual activities in their real lives. For a lot of women, fantasy can be a place of play that remains totally personal and private.

Justin Lehmiller, an American social psychologist, surveyed two thousand Americans about their fantasies and found a wide range in the frequency and content of fantasies. If you want to learn more about the kinds of fantasies everyday people have, I highly recommend his 2018 book *Tell Me What You Want*.

In our own mindfulness groups, women have shared that they sometimes fantasize about being with their partner but engaging in sexual activities they have never tried before or perhaps having sex in a new location. Sometimes they fantasize about being with a new lover or lovers. They fantasize about adopting a new identity. What makes fantasy exciting is that you can create a sexual scenario in your imagination that you will most probably never act on in real life. The ability to imagine is the key to enjoying the sexual benefits of fantasy.

If you have never tried to create a fantasy before, you might want to get a copy of one of Susie Bright's *Herotica* books or Emily Dubberley's *Garden of Desires: The Evolution of Women's Sexual*

Fantasies. These books are relatively inexpensive and are available at many bookstores and online. They all contain a variety of fantasies, some of which you might like more than others, and will give you an idea of the sheer range of fantasies. They might also help you feel more comfortable about exploring and creating your own fantasies. Some women like to share their fantasies with their partners. Others prefer to keep them private.

More recently there have been web-enabled programs as well as apps that deliver sexual fantasies to the listener through audio. One program, Dipsea, delivers short sexual stories that are relatable and feminist, with a focus on pleasure rather than performance. Many of our mindful sex participants have raved about Dipsea as a way of helping them tune in to the power of fantasy in a wholly permission-granting and shame-busting way.

Now that we have introduced fantasy and how it might be elicited, let's consider how fantasy can be used with mindfulness.

FORMAL EXERCISE 7: FANTASY PLUS SEXUAL SENSATIONS AWARENESS PRACTICE

In the following mindfulness exercise, you will use fantasy as a tool to elicit physical sexual sensations. Begin by checking in with what your thoughts and feelings are right now. What thoughts are present? How are you feeling? Then, for a few minutes, use all of your senses to evoke a vivid sexual fantasy. The more you can include your various senses, the more real the experience will feel for you. Try to tune in to smells, touches, and sounds. Your fantasy might include a few brief images instead of an entire scene, and that is fine. There might be more romantic components than explicitly sexual components, and that is fine too. This is all about you and what works for you. Maybe your fantasy is a memory of a wonderful sexual encounter from the past. Or maybe it is an entirely fictionalized scenario involving you and a new partner engaging in sexual activities you have never tried. Try to create a vivid image of yourself feeling comfortable with your sexuality. Remember that your fantasy is your own, and you can create it in whatever way is most pleasing to you.

If you prefer, you can read a fantasy from a book or listen to a fantasy from a web-enabled program or app. Take about ten minutes to fully attend to this fantasy and bring it to life in your imagination.

WHAT YOU WILL NEED

- A comfortable chair or bed
- A quiet space (remember that no space will be totally silent, and that is okay!)
- A fantasy of your choice
- Your journal

This practice will take about ten minutes.

STEP-BY-STEP GUIDE TO FANTASY PLUS SEXUAL SENSATIONS AWARENESS

- Lie in bed or sit on a comfortable chair in a relaxed position. Close your eyes. Elicit your fantasy.

- Once you have experienced sexual arousal in your mind and body, you are ready to set that fantasy aside and engage in this mindfulness practice.

- Focus on what is going on in your body right now. Observe your energy level, the sensations of breathing, and perhaps the sensations of your heart beating.

- Notice sensations on your skin, perhaps tingling, warmth, or coolness.

- Now bring your attention to your facial expressions and any sensations in your face.

- After a moment, move your focus of attention down your body, past your chest and belly, and down to your pelvis. Take a few breaths.

- Next, tune in to the sensations in your genitals. Allow your focus of attention to rest gently on your vulva and vagina. Notice the individual sensations in this area of your body, as each sensation emerges, lingers, and fades away. Become aware of how your genitals feel, moment to moment. There may be tingling, warmth, fullness, pulsating, or an absence of sensation. Just notice what is there.

- Notice if you experience the sensations in your genitals as pleasant, unpleasant, or neutral. If you like them, do you feel an urge to move toward them? If you dislike them, do you feel an urge to push them away? If they feel neutral to you, do you feel an urge to make those neutral feelings more pleasurable?

- Do you experience the sensations as sexual?

- Whenever you notice that you have forgotten about noticing sensations in your genitals because your attention was engaged in the content of a thought or a story, simply note where your attention has gone and gently return it to sensations in your genitals. Notice whatever is there in this moment.

- Next, try to narrow the focus of your attention to the different parts of your genitals. Notice sensations in the clitoris and the mons, or naturally hair-covered area, above the clitoris. Move the focus of your attention downward to the sensations in your labia. Notice the sensations at the vaginal entrance and inside the vagina. Spend some minutes there just observing with curiosity.

- Should judgments or thoughts arise, try to treat them in the same way as you would treat clouds floating by in a spacious sky. They can move past you and out of view so that you can return to focus on what is important now—your body.

- Expand the focus of your attention again to your genitals as a whole and allow your attention to move fluidly to whatever genital sensation is most vivid, moment to moment. Notice if you experience the sensations as pleasant, unpleasant, or neutral. Perhaps notice if you experience them as sexual. If so, how can you tell the sensations are sexual? Linger there for a few minutes, paying even closer attention to whatever sensations arise.

- Now, expand the focus of your attention around your genitals to include a sense of your body as a whole, lying here, breathing. Allow your attention to rest on whatever sensation is most prominent, moment to moment, wherever it is located in your body.

- Continue doing this for a few minutes.

- As you come to the end of this practice, congratulate yourself for taking this time to cultivate your awareness of sexual sensations in your body. And then, when you are ready, gently open your eyes.

- Finally, take a few deep breaths before you move on to the Inquiry.

THE INQUIRY

Spend the next ten to fifteen minutes reading and answering the three Inquiry questions. Again, you can say your answers aloud, write them down in your journal, or simply reflect on them. Whichever option you choose, though, take the time to consider each question in detail.

QUESTION 1. What did you notice during this practice?

Consider what sensations arose during this practice with a focus on the bare sensations. Can you describe them in detail? How long did each sensation last? How long did the following sensation last? What else came up for you as you paid attention to the sensations in your genitals specifically?

QUESTION 2. How was paying attention to your body and your genitals, in the way you just did, different from how you normally observe sensations in your body?

This exercise involved first engaging in a sexual fantasy and then paying attention to your body sensations. How was noticing the sensations in your body and in your genitals different from how you normally pay attention to feelings in those body parts? Try to be as detailed as possible.

QUESTION 3. How was this exercise relevant to your sexuality?

How was paying attention to the sensations in your body and in the different parts of your genitals after you had engaged in a fantasy relevant to your sexual desire or sexual arousal? What learnings can you take from this Fantasy plus Sexual Sensations Awareness practice to apply to your sexual health?

END OF THE FANTASY PLUS SEXUAL SENSATIONS AWARENESS PRACTICE

What was that exercise like for you? How vividly could you create a sexual fantasy in your mind, or, if you were reading or listening to one, how effectively did the story elicit a fantasy in your imagination? What did you notice in your body when you shifted to the Sexual Sensations Awareness practice? What kinds of sensations did you experience? How intense were they?

Tune in to the sensations that remain in your body after this exercise. Do you notice an increase in your heart rate? Does your skin feel different? Do you notice genital excitement?

If you think it would be helpful, write your thoughts down in your journal.

OTHER WAYS OF INCORPORATING FANTASY

You could also experiment with incorporating fantasy into sexual activity with your partner. You might decide to use fantasy while you are exploring your partner's body, or while you are having oral sex or vaginal penetration/intercourse with your partner. How and when you use fantasy is up to you.

Give yourself permission to experiment with fantasy. Mindfulness is about compassionate acceptance, and you have been cultivating that now for several weeks. Use that same self-compassion to allow yourself to try something new in this practice. If you do not like it, you can always discontinue it.

VIBRATORS: USING EXTERNAL PHYSICAL STIMULATION TO ELICIT SEXUAL AROUSAL

In the late 1800s, a diagnosis of "hysteria" was given to women who experienced a diffuse mix of anxiety, restlessness, fatigue, irritability, and heaviness in their abdomens. *Hysteria* means "uterus" in Greek, and the use of the term is rooted in the belief that such symptoms were caused by a wandering uterus. Stimulation of the vulva and clitoris by male doctors was found to relieve women of their hysteria by inducing what they called a *paroxysm*. You might know it as an orgasm. Medical professionals and the public alike thought that the release of tension through these paroxysms could treat women's hysteria, and women flocked to their male physicians' offices for treatment.

Eliciting a paroxysm by hand was inefficient (and tiring), however, and eventually the vibrator became the tool of choice to deliver this treatment. In 1880, an English physician named Sir Joseph Mortimer Granville invented the electromechanical vibrator as a tool to ease general muscle aches and pains. Within a short period of time, his vibrator had been adopted as a sexual health treatment tool, although it was marketed as a "personal massager." Over the years, women began to purchase their own electric, and eventually battery-operated, vibrators, thus omitting the need for a male physician to elicit the paroxysm on their behalf.

These days vibrators are marketed solely as a means of eliciting sexual pleasure. A large population-based survey from 2009 shows that 53 percent of women have tried a vibrator, and 31 percent have used them during sexual activity either alone or with a partner at least once in the past year.

A vibrator can be a helpful tool to increase or improve your natural sexual arousal response. If you do not own one, or you own one but you don't particularly like it, do some shopping around to find the right vibrator for you. Given the variety of shapes, sizes, intensities, and vibration patterns available, you might find it helpful to experiment with a few models before choosing one. You might wish to include your partner, if you have one, in your research. Look up the "adult stores" in your area and consider dropping by to view the products and speak with a staff member. In Vancouver, where I live, the adult stores are staffed by sex educators who are credible and reliable and provide excellent information about products and how to optimize your sexual health. Many pharmacies also carry vibrators and massagers in the contraceptive aisle.

Have you previously used a vibrator? What do you think about using one to create sexual pleasure? Read through the next exercise and think about how you feel about using one in it.

Some women are concerned that using a vibrator is an artificial way to experience sexuality and are therefore strongly against using them. If you share this belief, try to address it with compassion and self-acceptance as you do the next exercise. Allow yourself to consider the vibrator simply as another option for improving your experience of sex. Give yourself permission to experiment a little bit. If you do not like it, you can always put it away after this exercise.

FORMAL EXERCISE 8: VIBRATOR PLUS SEXUAL SENSATIONS AWARENESS PRACTICE

Start by checking in with what is going on for you right now. How are you feeling? Note any physical sensations in your body that are calling for your attention. What about mental sensations or emotions? Can you become aware of anything there? Take five deep breaths.

WHAT YOU WILL NEED

- A comfortable chair or bed
- A quiet space (remember that no space will be totally silent, and that is okay!)
- A vibrator of your choice
- Your journal

This practice will take about ten minutes plus a few minutes beforehand to use your vibrator. You will follow some of the same mindful practice instructions that you did in the Fantasy plus Sexual Sensations Awareness practice.

STEP-BY-STEP GUIDE TO VIBRATOR PLUS SEXUAL SENSATIONS AWARENESS PRACTICE

- Get to know your vibrator by turning it on and adjusting the settings, if it comes with settings. Place it on your thigh and close your eyes.

- Tune in to the sensations that begin to emerge. Take some time now to move it around to different parts of your body. Many vibrators are shaped like a penis, but most women place their vibrator on or close to their clitoris rather than inside their vagina. You can experiment by placing it in different locations.

- Notice all your sensations. Notice if any feelings of pleasure are beginning to emerge. Focus your attention on the sensation of touch.

- Closing your eyes can help you focus. Notice whether having your eyes closed has any effect on your physical sensations. If you wish to increase the intensity of the vibration, do so now. If you sense increasing tension in your body, just notice it. If you feel that you are getting close to orgasm, ease up on the intensity of the vibration and move the vibrator to a non-erotic part of your body.

- After a few minutes of using the vibrator to elicit your physical arousal, switch it off and set it aside as you move into the mindfulness practice.

- Lie in bed or sit on a comfortable chair in a relaxed position. Close your eyes, if that feels comfortable, and focus on what is going on in your body right now. Observe your energy level, the sensations of breathing, and perhaps the sensations of your heart beating.

- Notice sensations on your skin, perhaps tingling, warmth, or coolness.

- Now bring your attention to your facial expressions and any sensations in your face.

- After a moment, move your focus of attention down your body, past your chest and belly, and down to your pelvis. Take a few breaths.

- Next, tune in to the sensations in your genitals. Allow your focus of attention to rest gently on your vulva and vagina. Notice the individual sensations in this area of your body, as each sensation emerges, lingers, and fades away. Become aware of how your genitals feel, moment to moment. There may be tingling, warmth, fullness, pulsating, or an absence of sensation. Just notice what is there.

- Notice if you experience the sensations in your genitals as pleasant, unpleasant, or neutral. If you like them, do you feel an urge to move toward them? If you dislike them, do you feel an urge to push them away? If they feel neutral to you, do you feel an urge to make those neutral feelings more pleasurable?

- Do you experience the sensations as sexual?

- Whenever you notice that you have forgotten about noticing sensations in your genitals because your attention was engaged in the content of a thought or a story, simply note where your attention has gone and gently return it to sensations in your genitals. Notice whatever is there in this moment.

- Next, try to narrow the focus of your attention to the different parts of your genitals. Notice sensations in the clitoris and the mons, or naturally hair-covered area, above the clitoris. Move the focus of your attention downward to the sensations in your labia. Notice the sensations at the vaginal entrance and inside the vagina. Spend some minutes there just observing with curiosity.

- Should judgments or thoughts arise, try to treat them in the same way as you would treat clouds floating by in a spacious sky. They can move past you and out of view so that you can return to focus on what is important now—your body.

- Expand the focus of your attention again to your genitals as a whole and allow your attention to move fluidly to whatever genital sensation is most vivid, moment to moment. Notice if you experience the sensations as pleasant, unpleasant, or neutral. Perhaps notice if you experience them as sexual. If so, how can you tell the sensations are sexual? Linger there for a few minutes, paying even closer attention to whatever sensations arise.

- Now, expand the focus of your attention around your genitals to include a sense of your body as a whole, lying here, breathing. Allow your attention to rest on whatever sensation is most prominent, moment to moment, wherever it is located in your body.

- Continue doing this for a few minutes.

- As you come to the end of this practice, congratulate yourself for taking this time to cultivate your awareness of sexual sensations in your body. And then, when you are ready, gently open your eyes.

- Finally, take a few deep breaths before you move on to the Inquiry.

THE INQUIRY

Spend the next ten to fifteen minutes reading and answering the three Inquiry questions. You can say your answers aloud, write them down in your journal, or simply reflect on them. Whichever option you choose, though, take the time to consider each question in detail.

QUESTION 1. What did you notice during this practice?

Consider what sensations arose during this practice with a focus on the bare sensations. Can you describe those feelings in detail? How long did each sensation last? How long did the sensation following each one last? What else came up for you as you paid attention to the sensations in your genitals specifically?

QUESTION 2. How was paying attention to your body and your genitals, in the way you just did, different from how you normally observe sensations in your body?

This exercise involved first using a vibrator and then paying attention to your body sensations. How was noticing the sensations in your body and in your genitals different from how you normally pay attention to feelings in those body parts? Try to be as detailed as possible.

QUESTION 3. How was this exercise relevant to your sexuality?

How was paying attention to the sensations in your body and in the different parts of your genitals after you had used a vibrator relevant to your sexual desire or sexual arousal? What learnings can you take from this Vibrator plus Sexual Sensations Awareness practice to apply to your sexual health?

END OF THE VIBRATOR PLUS SEXUAL SENSATIONS AWARENESS PRACTICE

What was that exercise like for you? What kinds of sensations did you experience from using the vibrator alone? What did you notice in your body when you shifted to the sexual sensations awareness practice? What kinds of sensations did you sense? How intense were they?

Tune in to the sensations that remain in your body after this exercise. Do you notice an increase in your heart rate? Does your skin feel different? Do you notice tingling or lubrication in your genital area?

If it is helpful, write your thoughts in your journal.

OTHER WAYS OF INCORPORATING A
VIBRATOR TO ELICIT SEXUAL AROUSAL

In the exercise above, I invited you to use a vibrator to elicit sexual arousal and to stop before you reached orgasm. You then used your mindfulness skills to tune in to the feelings you elicited. If you already regularly use a vibrator, either with or without a partner, you might try to bring more mindfulness to your physical sensations while you are using it. You can also experiment with the same exercise but continue until you reach orgasm. You could then use the mindfulness exercise described above to sense the feelings in your body following orgasm. By really paying attention, some women can sense contractions of the uterus. You might also notice an intense peak of muscle tension followed by release in other muscles of your body. Over the next few weeks, you could try pairing the vibrator with a mindfulness exercise. Try to incorporate the mindfulness skills you have been cultivating in the past few weeks to notice the burst of sensations, moment by moment, as each arises, lingers, and fades away.

EROTICA: USING AUDIOVISUAL MATERIAL
TO ELICIT SEXUAL AROUSAL

"Erotica" refers to any artistic or literary form that depicts something sexual. It comes from the term "erotic," which means tending to arouse sexual desire, and can include erotic sculptures, books, and movies. In this section, erotica means audiovisual material.

Erotica must be distinguished from pornography, or porn, which usually refers to the explicit depiction of sexual behavior with the goal of eliciting sexual excitement. Porn is commercially available, easily accessible, often (though not always) has the male viewer in mind, and focuses on images that are maximally sexually arousing to facilitate orgasm and ejaculation. Erotica places less emphasis on orgasm as the goal and instead is intended to elicit pleasure, usually incorporates a story and character development, is more likely to depict a range of body types and sexual activities, and is often experienced by the viewer as more visually pleasing because the producers have put effort into using attractive décor, etc. Using erotica might help to increase your sexual arousal and help you to better understand what does and does not turn you on.

While much pornography is aimed at male viewers, you might be interested in exploring feminist pornography, which really increased in production in the mid-1980s. Candida Royalle, who worked as an actor in traditional pornographic films, branched off and developed Femme Productions, which sought to create pornography with female pleasure as the focal point. Feminist pornography became very popular around that time, and a number of other women were inspired to become producers and directors of this new art form. Female-friendly erotica is not as widely available as traditional porn and you might need to put in some time and effort to find it. In my own research program at the University of British Columbia, we have exclusively used "female-friendly erotica" for almost twenty years as a tool for eliciting sexual response in the laboratory, and then measuring the nature and intensity of sexual arousal that follows. During that time we have asked research participants for their preferences in erotica and as a result have greatly expanded our library of material.

What are your own feelings about audiovisual erotica? Do you have any experience with using it? Many women find themselves turned on when they hear a certain erotic story or watch a particular erotic scene. How do you feel if or when this happens? Many women have mixed feelings about their response to erotica, especially if they are morally or ethically against it. They often feel confused, embarrassed, or even ashamed when their body becomes aroused by it. If you can accept erotica as normal and healthy and view it as an occasional enhancer of sexual feelings, you might find it very helpful.

FORMAL EXERCISE 9: EROTICA PLUS SEXUAL SENSATIONS AWARENESS PRACTICE

Try to explore different forms of audiovisual erotica that you might find pleasing. You could choose erotic movies with female directors and more of a focus on the woman than you would find in what we might call traditional pornographic movies, which tend to be male-made and male-focused. Several women who have participated in our program have noted that the female-made, female-focused movies are less focused on heterocentric penile-vaginal intercourse and depict a broader array of arousing activities. In the following practice, you might choose to read through the instructions before you view your selected erotica.

After you have explored different erotic movies, select one for this practice. Check in with how you are feeling. What do you notice in your body? What kinds of thoughts are arising? Set any expectations aside and use this as an opportunity to really pay attention.

WHAT YOU WILL NEED

- A comfortable chair (a recliner is ideal) or bed
- A quiet space (remember that no space will be totally silent, and that is okay!)
- An erotic movie of your choice
- Your journal

This practice will take about ten minutes plus up to ten minutes of viewing erotica first. You will follow some of the same mindful practice instructions that you did in the Fantasy plus Sexual Sensations Awareness practice.

STEP-BY-STEP GUIDE TO EROTICA PLUS SEXUAL SENSATIONS AWARENESS PRACTICE

- Get into a comfortable position in your chair or bed and take a deep breath.

- Spend up to ten minutes watching the erotica you've selected.

- Turn off the movie and tune in to your body. Note what physical sensations emerge. Try to pay attention to subtle changes in how your genital area feels before you move into the mindfulness practice.

- Close your eyes, if that feels comfortable, and focus on what is going on in your body right now. Observe your energy level, the sensations of breathing, and perhaps the sensations of your heart beating.

- Notice sensations on your skin, perhaps tingling, warmth, or coolness.

- Now bring your attention to your facial expressions and any sensations in your face.

- After a moment, move your focus of attention down your body, past your chest and belly, and down to your pelvis. Take a few breaths.

- Next, tune in to the sensations in your genitals. Allow your focus of attention to rest gently on your vulva and vagina. Notice the individual sensations in this area of your body, as each sensation emerges, lingers, and fades away. Become aware of how your genitals feel, moment to moment. There may be tingling, warmth, fullness, pulsating, or an absence of sensation. Just notice what is there.

- Notice if you experience the sensations in your genitals as pleasant, unpleasant, or neutral. If you like them, do you feel an urge to move toward them? If you dislike them, do you feel an urge to push them away? If they feel neutral to you, do you feel an urge to make those neutral feelings more pleasurable?

- Do you experience the sensations as sexual?

- Whenever you notice that you have forgotten about noticing sensations in your genitals because your attention was engaged in the content of a thought or a story, simply note where your attention has gone and gently return it to sensations in your genitals. Notice whatever is there in this moment.

- Next, try to narrow the focus of your attention to the different parts of your genitals. Notice sensations in the clitoris and the mons, or naturally hair-covered area, above the clitoris. Move the focus of your attention downward to the sensations in your labia. Notice the sensations at the vaginal entrance and inside the vagina. Spend some minutes there just observing with curiosity.

- Should judgments or thoughts arise, try to treat them in the same way as you would treat clouds floating by in a spacious sky. They can move past you and out of view so that you can return to focus on what is important now—your body.

- Expand the focus of your attention again to your genitals as a whole and allow your attention to move fluidly to whatever genital sensation is most vivid, moment to moment. Notice if you experience the sensations as pleasant, unpleasant, or neutral. Perhaps notice if you experience them as sexual. If so, how can you tell the sensations are sexual? Linger there for a few minutes, paying even closer attention to whatever sensations arise.

- Now, expand the focus of your attention around your genitals to include a sense of your body as a whole, lying here, breathing.

Allow your attention to rest on whatever sensation is most prominent, moment to moment, wherever it is located in your body.

· Continue doing this for a few minutes.

· As you come to the end of this practice, congratulate yourself for taking this time to cultivate your awareness of sexual sensations in your body. And then, when you are ready, gently open your eyes.

· Finally, take a few deep breaths before you move on to the Inquiry.

THE INQUIRY

Spend the next ten to fifteen minutes reading and answering the three Inquiry questions. Again, you can say your answers aloud, write them down in your journal, or simply reflect on them. Whichever option you choose, though, take the time to consider each question in detail.

QUESTION 1. What did you notice during this practice?

Consider what sensations arose during this practice with a focus on the bare sensations. Can you describe those feelings in detail? How long did each sensation last? How long did the sensation following each one last? What else came up for you as you paid attention to the sensations in your genitals specifically?

QUESTION 2. How was paying attention to your body and your genitals, in the way you just did, different from how you normally observe sensations in your body?

This exercise involved first involved watching some erotica, and then paying attention to your body sensations. How was noticing the sensations in your body and in your genitals different from how you normally pay attention to feelings in those body parts? Try to be as detailed as possible.

QUESTION 3. How was this exercise relevant to your sexuality?

How was paying attention to the sensations in your body and in the different parts of your genitals after you had watched erotica relevant to your sexual desire or sexual arousal? What learnings can you take from this Erotica plus Sexual Sensations Awareness practice to apply to your sexual health?

END OF THE EROTICA PLUS SEXUAL SENSATIONS AWARENESS PRACTICE

What was that exercise like for you? What sensations did you notice while you were watching the erotica? How did those sensations change when you turned it off and did the mindfulness practice? What kinds of sensations did you sense? How intense were they? Where were they located?

Tune in to the sensations that remain in your body after this exercise. Do you notice an increase in your heart rate? Does your skin feel different? Do you notice genital sensations?

If it's helpful, write your thoughts in your journal.

RESOURCES FOR EROTIC TOOLS

Most bookstores have an erotic literature section where you can find a wide variety of novels and short stories, such as one of Susie Bright's Herotica books, or Garden of Desires: The Evolution of Women's Sexual Fantasies by Emily Dubberley, or Best Women's Erotica, edited by sex columnist Violet Blue. Your local public library may also have some. If you prefer fantasy books depicting scenes of dominance and submission, you may enjoy Please, Sir by J. A. Bailey and Yes, Sir by Rachel Kramer Bussel.

If you are looking for audiovisual erotica made by female directors, I recommend Erika Lust films (www.erikalust.com) and Candida Royalle films (www.candidaroyalle.com). Abby Winters films depict real couples having sex (www.abbywinters.com). Please use only ethically created audiovisual erotica. That means the actors are of legal age and are compensated appropriately for their acting.

Most cities around the world are home to at least one adult store, or sex toy store. The following have been highly recommended by my own mindful sex group participants:

· Pink Cherry: www.pinkcherry.ca (Oakville, Ontario, Canada)
· Come As You Are: www.comeasyouare.com (click on Sex Info for accurate information about sexual enhancement products) (Toronto, Ontario, Canada)
· Little Shop of Pleasures: www.littleshopofpleasures.com (Calgary, Alberta, Canada)
· Womyns' Ware: www.womynsware.com (Vancouver, British Columbia, Canada)
· The Art of Loving: www.artofloving.ca (Vancouver, British Columbia, Canada)

STRUGGLES AND STRATEGIES

The struggles covered below are related to staying present during sexual activity; the Sexual Sensations Awareness practices involving fantasy, vibrators, and erotica; and the process of acquiring a vibrator or erotica. If you feel the strategies below would not work for you, feel free to add your own.

THE STRUGGLE: AS MUCH AS I TRY TO PAY ATTENTION DURING SEXUAL ACTIVITY, IT IS JUST TOO CHALLENGING. Minds are busy. Even though you might start a sexual encounter feeling "present," you might find that your mind easily drifts away, enticed by distractions or even judgments. The beginning of this chapter includes suggestions for how you can use your senses to "bring you back" to the present moment during sex, but you might find that these strategies are not working in the way you hoped.

Strategies

- Be patient. You've likely spent many years inadvertently perfecting the art of distraction and you now move into it automatically. Deliberately paying attention during sex might be very new to you and, like all skills, it will require some practice.

- Become aware of whether there are particular days, times, settings, or locations that make it easier for you to bring mindfulness into sexual activity. Plan sexual activity for the times when you find it easier to be and remain present.

- Be compassionate toward yourself when you get distracted during sex. If you judge yourself for struggling to remain present, that judgment can contribute to further disconnection from the present moment. Some people find doing a brief compassion meditation before or even at the start of sexual activity can allow them to go into the encounter with openness to and acceptance of whatever might arise. Tara Brach has some excellent, free, and downloadable compassion meditations at www.tarabrach.com.

THE STRUGGLE: I AM TOO EMBARRASSED TO GO INTO A STORE TO PURCHASE A VIBRATOR.

Taboos continue to surround women's sexuality, despite today's seemingly sex-saturated society, and this might make you feel embarrassed about purchasing a vibrator. You might worry about being seen by someone who knows you, for example.

Strategies

- It is highly unlikely you will see someone you know at the precise moment you decide to go into a store to buy a vibrator.

- Use humor. If you do see someone you know, laugh it off by saying something like, "Wow, this is awkward!" or "Is this too much information?" or even "Fancy seeing you here!"

- Consider purchasing a vibrator online. Most of the adult stores that sell high-quality vibrators have an online purchasing option and their products are delivered in discreet packaging.

- Consider leaning in to your embarrassment and using mindfulness to identify the sensations in your body. Tuning in is far more effective than tuning out.

THE STRUGGLE: I FEEL BAD WHEN I ELICIT A FANTASY.
As I described earlier in this chapter, many people have said that their fantasy does not match what they do or want to do in their real-life sex lives.

Strategies

- You do not need to enact the fantasy in your real life. You created it in your mind and you can keep it there.

- Remember that no one needs to know that you are engaging in a fantasy.

- Try engaging in a fantasy while you work through this workbook. If it is not for you, you can set it aside once you complete this workbook.

TIME TO PRACTICE

Over the next week, if you plan to be sexually active, try to engage each of your senses in the present moment as a way of practicing mindful sex. This will be your informal practice for the week. If this is the first time you are practicing mindfulness during sexual activity, you might want to start with one sense (e.g., touch) and then move on to another one (e.g., sight) before trying to integrate awareness of all your senses during the encounter. If you are engaging in sexual activity with a partner, you may or may not elect to tell them that you are practicing mindful sex. You might choose to explain it to them, or show them the instructions at the start of this chapter and practice it together. You might offer to slow down considerably to allow both of you time to really tune in to the present. You might also choose to not tell your partner that you're integrating mindfulness into sex but keep it to yourself. That is fine too.

Try the Sexual Sensations Awareness practice with any of the sexual tools I discussed: fantasy, vibrator, or erotica. Or you can try all three (one at a time!). Again, the invitation is to first engage with the sexual tool for approximately ten minutes, or as much time as it takes to elicit a small amount of sexual arousal, but before orgasm. You would then set the sexual tool aside and either read or listen to the Sexual Sensations Awareness practice.

If there are any practices from previous chapters that you have not tried yet, try to find time to practice them this week before you move on to chapter 7.

7
Aversion and Attachment

WHAT ARE AVERSION AND ATTACHMENT?

Throughout our mindfulness practices so far, I've invited you to pay attention to your bodily sensations and to notice whether you like or dislike them. During the first mindfulness exercise, which involved eating a piece of food, you may have wanted to prolong the pleasant feelings you experienced while you were eating slowly, or you may have wanted the more unpleasant sensations you experienced from eating slowly to end.

Let's consider this a bit more deeply. Every physical and mental sensation is associated with a feeling or tone of pleasant, unpleasant, or neutral (that is, neither pleasant nor unpleasant), as you have likely noticed by now. When pleasant sensations arise, a common reaction is to want to stay with those sensations and often to engage in thoughts or actions to create more of them.

In contrast, when unpleasant sensations arise, we habitually pull away or even react with aversion, attempting to push the unpleasant sensation away. This pushing away can be accompanied by physical tension somewhere in the body as well as thoughts and actions we think will cause the unpleasant sensations to stop. When neutral sensations arise, the tendency is to ignore them. If neutral sensations continue to arise for a prolonged period, we habitually react with aversion, engaging in thoughts and actions that attempt to push away the uninteresting, neutral sensations and replace them with something more interesting and ideally something pleasant. These habitual attachment and aversion reactions to transient sensations are the foundation of the basic unsatisfactoriness of our existence.

Although the pleasant, unpleasant, or neutral feeling associated with each sensation is not within our control, dissatisfaction or suffering only occurs if attachment or aversion to those feelings arises. As you continue to practice mindfulness, you gain firsthand experience and understanding of unsatisfactoriness. This will help you to accept unpleasant sensations, without necessarily needing to do anything to change them, and enjoy pleasant sensations, without necessarily needing to do anything to hold on to them. Eventually you will be able to experience pleasant, unpleasant, and neutral sensations just as they are without any need to avoid or cling to them. Sensations can then be seen as arising and then passing away in a process that can simply be observed, rather than needing to be changed.

In our practices so far, I've guided you to notice your physical and mental sensations. In the remaining mindfulness practices, I will also guide you to pay attention to your feelings of attachment and aversion to those bare sensations. In other words, you will be paying attention to both the sensations you experience and your reactions (i.e., attachment and aversion) to them.

HOW ARE AVERSION AND ATTACHMENT RELEVANT TO SEXUALITY?

During sexual activity do you ever want to change how you are feeling? For example, if you feel sexual arousal but it starts to fade, you may want to feel that arousal again and become frustrated if it continues to subside. You may try to push away your negative feelings of frustration or to cling to pleasant feelings, but these attempts can pull you into your head and further disconnect you from your sexual arousal and desire. How do you think this can affect your sexual feelings and sexual satisfaction?

Ultimately, you can reduce distress by accepting pleasant, unpleasant, and neutral sensations equally rather than trying to hold on to the pleasant ones and pushing away or changing the unpleasant or neutral ones. This is called equanimity, and it can be developed over time through mindfulness practices. Every time that you have tried to observe negative feelings, pain, or distressing memories from a distance and with acceptance in your practice, you have been practicing equanimity. You do not need to aim for full equanimity to reduce distress. Simply remembering to be mindful of all sensations—pleasant, unpleasant, or neutral— to see their impermanence in the moment, and to understand that sensations are just sensations, no more and no less important than any other feelings, will help to alleviate distress.

Most of the discussion up to this point has been about pleasant and unpleasant sensations, but what about the neutral ones? Sometimes, there are neutral (or no) sensations during sexual activity. Years ago, when I was working with gynecologic cancer survivors, many of them told me that they "felt nothing" when they or their partners touched their vulvas. In the past, stimulation there had been pleasurable, leading to mounting feelings of arousal and eventually orgasm. But after their treatments, they told me that all they felt was a hand against their skin. They did not experience any associated pleasurable feelings as they had in the past. In other words, they felt neutral. Part of our mindful sex approach during group work involved first practicing observing what neutral felt like, accepting it, and then moving on to doing exercises that might elicit a sexual response. In other words, accepting neutrality was a key part of their sexual rehabilitation.

Do you believe that sex should always be positive? Or that your partner "should" know how to arouse you? Or that all encounters should lead to orgasm? Are all encounters likely to be entirely pleasurable? Is that a realistic expectation? We know that having fixed expectations like these can result in disappointment and distress, which can directly impede sexual desire and response.

Could you imagine bringing equanimity to neutral feelings during sexual activity? And if so, how might this impact your overall sexual experience by having this openness to neutral feelings?

Take some time to think about these questions and then write your reflections about them in your journal.

FORMAL EXERCISE 10: WORKING WITH SENSATIONS IN THE BODY PRACTICE

In this practice, we will work with the concepts of aversion and attachment as I guide you to pay attention to all sensations—pleasant, unpleasant, and neutral. When you notice yourself clinging to good feelings, or wanting to turn off or avoid bad feelings, you will have the opportunity to practice equanimity and maintain the same openness to all sensations.

WHAT YOU WILL NEED

- A chair, ideally high-back
- A quiet space (remember that no space will be totally silent, and that is okay!)
- Comfortable socks or shoes
- Your journal

This practice will take about fifteen minutes.

STEP-BY-STEP GUIDE TO WORKING WITH SENSATIONS IN THE BODY

- Find a position in your chair that promotes a state of relaxed wakefulness. Thank yourself for taking this time to take care of yourself by doing this mindfulness practice. When you are ready, gently close your eyes, or if you prefer, rest your gaze softly on a fixed spot in front of you.

- Begin by letting your body find its own natural, comfortable position. Find a position and posture that promote comfort in your spine. Your eyes and face should be soft and your shoulders relaxed and comfortable.

- Focus your attention on the sensations of breathing, in whatever region they are most vivid for you in this moment—perhaps the belly, the chest, or the nostrils. Feel the sensations of the in-breath and of the out-breath, not changing your breath, just allowing your body to breathe by itself.

- You may, of course, have thoughts drifting through your mind—for example, memories of conversations you had earlier in the day, or thoughts about planning the rest of your day. Simply acknowledge whatever is there.

- Do your best to stay alert and mentally focused throughout the practice.

- Whenever a physical sensation in another area of your body, a sound, or a thought becomes predominant, momentarily take this to be the new focus for attention, and bring the same level of mindful awareness to that sensation, sound, or thought, continuing to observe it until it is no longer predominant. Then bring your attention back to your breath and to the region of your body you are focusing on.

- Move even closer to the individual sensations that make up your in-breath and your out-breath. Notice the slight pause in between the in-breath and the out-breath, and between the out-breath and the next in-breath.

- Notice the individual qualities of your breath, perhaps coolness or warmth, swirling or whooshing sensations. Notice tingling, tightness, itching, pressure, or whatever else is there.

- Observe the individual breath sensations as they emerge, linger, and fade away.

- Whenever you notice that you have forgotten about noticing your breath sensations because your attention was engaged in or identifying with the content of a thought, notice what your attention was engaged with and then, with kindness, return your attention to the sensations of breathing in the region you are focusing on. Without any judgment or blame, just begin again.

- Use your breath as an anchor to gently reconnect with the here-and-now.

- As you sit and focus on your breath, if any strong sensations arise in other parts of your body—tingling, pain, itchiness, tension—just take note that they are there. Whenever those sensations are more prominent than your breath sensations, release your focus on your breath and focus on those strong sensations until they no longer dominate, and then return the focus of your attention to the sensations of breathing.

- Now, expand your focus of attention on your breath to include your body as a whole. Allow your attention to move fluidly from sensation to sensation as each emerges, lingers, and fades away.

- As you are paying attention in this way, try to receive all sensations with friendliness and kindness. Perhaps name strong sensations—for example, hot, itching, or pain. Move even closer to the sensations. Bring an equal interest and curiosity to all sensations as they arise, whether they are pleasant, unpleasant, or neutral.

- When any strong sensations subside, refocus your attention on the sensations of breathing.

- In the next few breaths, pay attention to the follow-on thoughts or reactions after you notice an initial strong sensation.

- If you feel discomfort, tension, restlessness, or irritation anywhere in your body, notice if you have any follow-on reactions to that. Do you want to end the discomfort or tension?

- How do you experience that aversion, that wanting an uncomfortable sensation to end? Where do you feel the aversion in your body? If it starts to subside, refocus your attention on the sensations themselves. Then notice the aversion again if it arises.

- Notice the bare sensations themselves when they are the most predominant, and notice the follow-on reactions when they are the most predominant.

- Next, begin to pay attention to neutral sensations, not just a lack of sensation, but sensations that are present in your body that you experience as neither pleasant nor unpleasant. Just neutral.

- Begin now to observe your neutral sensations—a mild tingling or a subtle awareness of a particular body part, an awareness of your spine as you hold your body upright, perhaps blood flow in some region of your body, saliva in your mouth, or the sensation of swallowing, or even the movement of air through your nostrils or into or out of your lungs.

- Begin to notice follow-on thoughts or reactions attached to these neutral sensations. How do you experience or perceive them? Do you wish for a stronger sensation, either pleasant or unpleasant, to focus on? Do you have a tendency to ignore or not pay attention to neutral sensations? Or do you appreciate neutral sensations after previously paying attention to unpleasant sensations? Or maybe you find yourself searching for a different sensation to focus on? Notice where these sensations show up in your body and if you observe other sensations associated with them—a sense of restlessness or contentment or some other sensation.

- Move back and forth between noticing the sensations and then observing your reactions to them.

- Now shift toward pleasant sensations. If you notice a place in your body where there is some comfort, relaxation, coziness, warmth, or pleasant tingling, for example, notice first of all the sensations that make up those pleasant sensations. And notice any follow-on reactions to your recognition of them. Do you wish for them to continue or feel an attachment to your good feelings? Do you notice a desire to not move away from focusing on that area? Where do you feel that attachment in your body? And if the attachment starts to subside, refocus your attention on the sensations themselves. When a feeling of attachment arises again, notice what that feels like. Move back and forth between noticing the sensations and observing your reactions to the sensations.

- Whenever you notice that your attention has become unfocused or is engaged in the content of a thought or story, you can always come back to the sensations of breathing. When you are ready to come back, once again expand the focus of your attention on your breath to include sensations throughout your whole body. Allow your attention to move fluidly from sensation to sensation as each emerges, lingers, and fades away. The pleasant ones and the unpleasant ones. Just be present in this moment, welcoming all of the sensations that are there.

- Finally, try to narrow your focus of attention onto the sensations of breathing, in whatever region they are most vivid in this moment. Whenever your attention moves to a sensation elsewhere in your body, to a sound or a thought that is more prominent, allow that to be the focus of attention until it no longer predominates. At that point, you can move your attention back to your breath.

- Open your eyes, and while remaining fully aware of the present moment, read the following poem, twice:

  The Guest House

  This being human is a guest house.
  Every morning a new arrival.

  A joy, a depression, a meanness,
  some momentary awareness comes
  as an unexpected visitor.

  Welcome and entertain them all!
  Even if they are a crowd of sorrows,
  who violently sweep your house empty of its furniture,
  still, treat each guest honorably.
  He may be clearing you out
  for some new delight.

  The dark thought, the shame, the malice.
  Meet them at the door laughing and invite them in.

  Be grateful for whatever comes.
  Because each has been sent as a guide from beyond.

  —Jellaluddin Rumi. Translation by Coleman Barks

- Now form the intention to invite very subtle movements into your toes, and pay attention to the sensations that are elicited as your toes begin to gently move. Notice whether you experience those sensations as pleasant, unpleasant, or neutral.

- Next, form the intention to bring some movement into your fingertips. Notice whether you experience these sensations as pleasant, unpleasant, or neutral.

- Finally, take a few deep breaths before you move on to the Inquiry.

THE BETTER SEX THROUGH MINDFULNESS WORKBOOK

THE INQUIRY

Consider each of the following three questions. As you read these questions, spend time reflecting on the answers or write your answers down in your journal.

QUESTION 1. What did you notice during this practice of paying attention to sensations and to the follow-on feelings of attachment (toward pleasant sensations) and aversion (to unpleasant sensations)?

Although this is not the first mindfulness practice in which you paid attention to pleasant, unpleasant, and neutral sensations, you spent more time observing your follow-on thoughts and feelings after you noticed those sensations during this practice than in earlier practices. What did you notice? Were you as likely to experience attachment as you were to feel aversion? Did you spend more time observing one over the other?

What about observing neutral feelings? What was that like? And what were the follow-on thoughts and feelings as you observed neutral feelings?

Take your time in answering these questions. They are challenging.

QUESTION 2. How was paying attention to pleasant, unpleasant, and neutral sensations and then noticing the follow-on attachment and aversion feelings different from how you might usually relate to sensations?

You may have noticed during this practice that when you paid attention to pleasant, unpleasant, and neutral sensations they were temporary. How was this different from how you normally experience pleasant, unpleasant, and neutral sensations in your day-to-day life? By this time you may be aware that sensing these feelings as pleasant or unpleasant is normal and unavoidable, but you may still have a tendency to want to avoid the unpleasant feelings and to want to hold on to the pleasant ones.

QUESTION 3. How was this practice of observing neutral sensations and also paying attention to attachment and aversion relevant to your sexuality?

Sometimes sexual activity is associated with neutral feelings, which are neither pleasant nor unpleasant. In this practice you brought the same awareness and compassion to those neutral feelings as you did to the pleasant and unpleasant ones. How might this skill (of equanimity) be useful for improving your own sexuality? Can you imagine bringing equanimity to those times during sex when pleasure has waned and you feel nothing? Can relating to those sensations with the same openness with which you relate to the positive feelings help to reduce judgments about yourself and your sexuality? How else might this practice of noticing aversion be useful to you during sex?

Have you read "The Guest House" before today? The guest house is a metaphor for human experience, in which we often experience unwanted thoughts and emotions that can feel like intruders. When this happens, we resist having those unpleasant thoughts and emotions. We feel invaded when guests arrive without an invitation and try to distract ourselves from them.

"The Guest House" encourages us to practice equanimity with all of the guests, to "treat each guest honorably." This means that we bring the same kindness, compassion, and awareness to the invited guests (feelings of joy, excitement, anticipation) as we do to the uninvited ones, the intruders (depression, anxiety, sorrow, guilt, shame). In order to treat all the guests equally, we must accept them all, regardless of their emotional tone (and the distress that each of them may bring). We cannot pick and choose the feelings we want to pay attention to and "forget the rest." Instead, by bringing kindness and compassion to all of our emotions, thoughts, and sensations, we can help distress, suffering, and aversion fade. This practice of welcoming all of the guests essentially eliminates suffering.

How could the message of "The Guest House" be helpful in the context of your sexuality? Are there times during sex when you feel joy, elation, and frustration at the same time? When you do, what happens? Do you tend to focus only on the frustration and try to eliminate it? And then what happens to the joy and elation? Could you imagine trying to treat all of these emotional "guests" that arise during sex the same? What might the outcome be?

Rumi suggests that we should be grateful for whatever guests arrive. What? Be grateful for the frustration, sadness, guilt, and anxieties that might arise during sex? How can expressing an attitude of gratitude to these negative feelings during sex be helpful?

Write your reflections on this practice, as well as your answers to the questions posed above, in your journal.

END OF THE WORKING WITH SENSATIONS IN THE BODY PRACTICE

You've just completed a practice in which you spent more time than ever before focusing on pleasant, unpleasant, and neutral sensations. You tried to observe your attachment to positive sensations and aversion to negative sensations. And you tried to practice equanimity toward everything that came up for you. This was a challenging practice, so give yourself lots of compassion if you struggled. You might still find it difficult to imagine how paying attention to unpleasant feelings and aversion and welcoming negative feelings could possibly be helpful to your sex life.

Here are some comments participants have made after they completed the Working with Sensations in the Body practice in our groups:

- I do not usually pay attention to attachment and aversion. But this practice allowed me to see them at play and to watch them from a distance without getting too attached to them.

- I was surprised that pleasant and unpleasant feelings were so transient! I think usually I feel like they last forever, especially unpleasant ones.

- Even a neutral sensation is something for me to notice. Neutral does not mean absent, and this practice has allowed me to be attuned to those moments during sex when, yeah, things are just neutral.

- By accepting neutral feelings, I can see how useful that would be to my sex life for those moments when I lose arousal and all that is left is touch without pleasure. Maybe my striving to fix it is actually getting in the way of accessing that arousal again.

- During sex, as soon as I have one bad thought or feeling, it derails me! It pulls me away from any ongoing positive thoughts or feelings. I want my body to be like a guest house during sex, and this means welcoming all feelings, whether they are good or bad or neutral.

- I specifically want to practice equanimity of my experience during a sexual encounter. I can see that being very useful.

- Knowing that unpleasant sensations can be temporary and transient is very useful for me to know during sex because when those feelings come up, I can say to myself, "This will pass."

EDUCATION ABOUT SEX

INFORMAL EXERCISE: SELF-EVALUATION

In this exercise, you will read a series of statements and then pause to observe what images, thoughts, feelings, and physical sensations arise. The goal of this exercise is to help you become more aware of your own evaluations of your sexuality.

1. *I am a somewhat sexual woman.*
   Pause for a minute with your eyes closed. Pay attention to what comes up.

2. *I am not much of a sexual woman.*
   Pause for a minute with your eyes closed. Pay attention to what comes up.

3. *I am broken sexually.*
   Pause for a minute with your eyes closed. Pay attention to what comes up.

What came up for you as you read each of these statements? Did any emotions come up? Did you feel sad or depressed? Did you notice a deep pang or throbbing in your body? Did you feel tension anywhere? Did you rebel against the more negative statements and instead want to give a more positive message? Write your answers to these questions in your journal.

Statements like the ones above can cause us to feel bad about ourselves or get caught up in an unproductive argument with ourselves. Do these statements, or similar ones, ever surface in your own life?

Read the next three statements. As before, notice what feelings, thoughts, and sensations arise after you read each one.

1. *I am a somewhat sexual woman.*
   Pause for a minute with your eyes closed. Pay attention to what comes up.

2. I am a fairly sexual woman.

Pause for a minute with your eyes closed. Pay attention to what comes up.

3. I am a fully sexual, sensual woman.

Pause for a minute with your eyes closed. Pay attention to what comes up.

What came up as you read this set of statements? Did your feelings differ from when you read the first set of three statements? If so, in what way? Did you sense any opposition or resistance to these statements? Or perhaps you noticed you identified in some way or to some degree with them? Write your responses to these questions in your journal.

The way that we talk to ourselves has a significant effect on how we feel. The Cognitive Behavioral Model (a well-researched theory and system of therapy that highlights the relationships between our thoughts, feelings, and behaviors) showed us almost a hundred years ago that our thoughts affect our emotions and our behaviors. And each of those reciprocally affects the others. It is common to have moments of self-doubt about your sexuality and negative thoughts about, for example, your body image, sexual skills, or ability to respond sexually. But persistent negative thoughts and self-talk can directly and dramatically affect feelings such as anxiety, sadness, guilt, shame, anger, irritability, frustration, and resentment.

Throughout this workbook we have been practicing mindfulness of thoughts, and by now you have probably spent a lot of time "on the bank of the stream," watching your thoughts pass by without you jumping into the water and getting wet. You can now observe your thoughts from a distance and even identify them as worries or memories or plans without getting caught up in their content and pulled into a cascade of further thoughts. Now let us apply this same mindfulness of thoughts to your self-judgments about sex. We will practice letting them be, which is not the same as letting them go. Letting them go implies a deliberate attempt to push away these self-judgments. Instead you will invite them into your awareness, as "The Guest House" suggests. Meet them at the door laughing. And bring equanimity to those judgmental thoughts about sex that you bring to all your other thoughts.

At the same time, I want to encourage you to find a positive sexual statement that resonates for you. If "I am fully sexual" feels like too far a stretch, choose something softer and more realistic. Women in our mindful sex groups have "tried on" a variety of different positive mental images until they found one or two that they could relate to most. For example, a breast cancer survivor tried on "I am a sex goddess" and felt that it empowered her to address negative thoughts about sex when they surfaced. Although she did not truly believe that she was a "sex goddess," she loved being able to try on that identity and use it to benefit her sexuality when she chose.

Over the next week, I encourage you to note any time you have negative thoughts about your sexuality, your sexual performance, or your sexual function. Try to bring mindful acceptance to those judgments and let them be. Try to imagine your own guest house where such evaluations can enter alongside all the positive thoughts you have about yourself. They can coexist.

FORMAL EXERCISE 11:
PLEASURABLE SENSATIONS PRACTICE

The Pleasurable Sensations practice builds on the Sexual Sensations Awareness practices you did in chapter 6. The intention of those practices was to elicit a sexual arousal response assisted by various sexual tools—fantasy, a vibrator, and then erotica. I hope by now you have practiced one or more of those exercises at least once. If not, try to do so before proceeding to the Pleasurable Sensations practice below. In fact, you might want to try the Sexual Sensations Awareness exercise three times—once with each sexual tool—before doing this next exercise.

At the beginning of this chapter you did a mindfulness practice that allowed you to notice self-judgments and your attachments and aversions to them. You then practiced letting them be before moving on to a self-evaluation exercise to help you see how holding judgmental views about your sexuality can affect your emotions. The Pleasurable Sensations exercise draws on these self-evaluations in a positive way. After you have completed it, you will practice the Sexual Sensations meditation again.

Unlike the previous mindfulness exercises, the Pleasurable Sensations one is *goal-oriented*. You will deliberately evoke a positive image of yourself as a sexual person, then use one of your erotic tools to do the Sexual Sensations Awareness practice. In chapter 6 you just observed whatever came up. Now, by evoking a positive sexual image first, you will specifically be looking for signs of arousal and pleasure. That is what makes this exercise goal-oriented.

This practice will give you an opportunity to reconnect with sexual pleasure, something that may have been lost or diminished or buried for some time. For this exercise you might want to have a lubricant handy. You will also need one of the sexual tools discussed at length in chapter 6—a fantasy, a vibrator, or erotica.

There is an important feedback loop from your genitals to your brain, so as you notice physical sexual arousal during the mindfulness exercise, try to let those sensations register in your mind. It will interpret these sensations as sexual, which will increase your physical arousal.

WHAT YOU WILL NEED

· A comfortable chair or bed
· A quiet space (remember that no space will be totally silent, and that is okay!)
· An erotic tool of your choice—a fantasy, a vibrator, or erotica
· Your journal

Allow approximately fifteen minutes for this practice. You may want to select a time when you feel good about yourself, when there are few distractions, and when you are unlikely to be interrupted. If you wish to proceed to orgasm after completing this exercise, it is fine to do so.

STEP-BY-STEP GUIDE TO PLEASURABLE SENSATIONS MEDITATION

Step 1: Cultivate an image of yourself as a sexual woman.
· Imagine that you are a sexual, sensual woman who enjoys her sexuality and is fully capable of a healthy sexual response. You might tell yourself that you are a sexual woman or describe to yourself who you want to be sexually. Or you could conjure up a memory of your past sexual self and hold that vividly in your mind. You do not have to totally believe in that image of yourself in the moment. You are simply trying this identity on. You do not need to keep it on after you have completed this exercise.

Step 2: Use a sexual tool to activate your sexual response.
· If you have chosen to use a fantasy, close your eyes and spend ten minutes fantasizing about a sexual scene. If you are the actor in the fantasy, remind yourself of your positive sexual image as you take part in various activities. If you are imagining someone other than yourself in the fantasy, hold on to your own positive sexual image throughout.

- If you have chosen erotica or a vibrator as your sexual tool, receive the sensations they produce through the lens of your new sexual self-image. Continue using your sexual tool for about ten minutes but stop before you reach orgasm.

Step 3: Cultivate an awareness of sexual sensations.

- Gently close your eyes and focus your attention on any physical sensations.

- Starting at your feet, notice the point at which they touch the surface beneath you.

- Focus your attention on any sensations in your feet. Wiggle your toes and take note of what that feels like. Move the focus of your attention up to your ankles, calves, and knees, noticing any sensations, tension, or tingling and the temperature there. Spend a few moments on each body part as you move up your body.

- Next, focus your attention on your genitals. Imagine to yourself that you are sexy and fully capable of sexual response as you focus on this part of your body. Are you aware of any sensations in your labia, clitoris, or vagina? Notice if these sensations feel sexual. Contract your vaginal muscles and notice if that gives you a heightened sense of pleasure. Focus on the sensations produced in your genitals and take note of any thoughts or emotions that emerge.

- Remind yourself that these are important parts of your body and that they are closely involved in sexual pleasure and activity. They are yours.

- Whenever you become aware that you have forgotten about noticing the sensations in your genitals because you were engaged with the content of a thought or story, congratulate yourself on becoming aware of that. Notice what your attention had been engaged with and then gently and kindly return it to the sensations in your genitals at this moment.

- Move your hands to your genitals. While imagining to yourself that you are a sexual, sensual woman, lightly press your fingers on the area of your clitoris. Press on the area of your clitoral shaft and hood and then down each side of your outer labia. Lightly touch your inner labia. Notice how different amounts of pressure produce different sensations. Describe the sensations to yourself. Remind yourself that the goal of this exercise is to enhance your awareness of pleasurable sexual sensations. Move your fingers down to touch the outer entrance of your vagina, and then when you are ready, put some lubricant onto one or more fingers and move them inside.

- Describe your sensations to yourself. Contract your vaginal muscles and notice what that feels like with your finger or fingers inside.

- If you notice that you are thinking about the sensations or lack of sensations rather than experiencing them, gently and kindly redirect your attention to the sensations themselves.

- Next, if you feel comfortable, move the focus of your attention and your hands to the rest of your upper body, including your breast/chest area.

- Describe the sensations to yourself as you touch these parts of your body.

- Keep that positive sexual identity activated as you notice signs of pleasure in these parts of your body.

- For the next few minutes, allow your attention to move fluidly to all of the different physical feelings that you are experiencing while maintaining the image of yourself as a sexual and sensual woman. Don't worry if this image is hard to believe in this moment. Remember, you are just trying it on.

· If you notice negative thoughts, just note them ("Ah, judgmental thoughts are here") and, when they have faded away, redirect your attention to your bodily sensations. Do not be hard on yourself if you find this difficult.

· Continue for a few more moments before moving your hand away.

· Take five deep breaths as you thank your positive sexual image for being here with you.

· Open your eyes and rest for a few moments in awareness of your experience.

END OF THE PLEASURABLE SENSATIONS PRACTICE

This exercise combined three elements: (1) creating an image of yourself as a sexual woman, (2) eliciting sexual sensations by using an erotic tool, and (3) cultivating an awareness of sexual sensations by observing these activated sensations. What was that like for you? What physical sensations did you experience? What emotions surfaced? Was it challenging to identify and hold on to an image of yourself as sexual? Which one did you choose? How were the feelings of arousal in your body different in this exercise from those in the sexual sensations awareness meditation that you did in chapter 6? Record your reflections in your journal.

BEING GOAL-ORIENTED

If you are thinking to yourself that this was not a mindfulness exercise, you are correct! In the first step, to activate a positive sexual image, you used a method known as a *cognitive schema elicitation*, in which you conjure up a different view of yourself from how you usually see yourself. You probably do not see yourself as sexual all, or even most, of the time, but by temporarily becoming someone who is sexual and using a sexual tool, you may have felt increasing levels of arousal and a desire for orgasm. This is called being goal-oriented. Having a goal during sex is not inherently a bad thing. However, when people get too caught up in their goal, they narrow their focus on the finish line and miss out on the entire journey. For that reason, mindfulness was featured in the last step of the exercise to guide you to notice all of the activated sensations, including your desire to achieve a goal, if that came up for you.

Here are some comments participants in our groups have shared with me after this exercise:

· I surprised myself that I could try on such a positive sexual image of myself during this exercise even though I do not believe that about myself at all! It was fun to be someone else who had a robust sexuality!

· I definitely noticed an effect from the sexual self-image exercise during both the fantasy part of this exercise and the mindfulness part. During my fantasy, I was imagining myself as this sexual, sensual woman engaged in an amazing sexual encounter. Then when I did the sexual sensations meditation, I held on to this image of myself, and all the sensations in my body just seemed so intense!

· I had to remind myself a few times during the sexual self-image elicitation that it was okay to try this on, even though I did not believe it. And I think it made a difference.

· What a powerful exercise pairing self-imagery plus an erotic aid plus mindfulness! I want to practice this again and again.

· How do I involve my partner in this exercise?

STRUGGLES AND STRATEGIES

The struggles covered below are related to dealing with feelings of aversion and attachment. Think about which of these strategies you think would work for you. Which ones wouldn't work? Write some other possible strategies in your journal.

THE STRUGGLE: WHEN I SENSE AVERSION TO AN UNPLEASANT SENSATION, I JUST WANT TO MOVE AWAY FROM IT. IT IS SO CHALLENGING TO BRING MINDFULNESS TO AVERSION.

It is natural for us to move away from or want to ignore unpleasant sensations and the aversion that follows the unpleasant sensations. You are not alone if you feel this way.

Strategies

· Because cultivating equanimity is an important part of an established mindfulness practice, try to reassure yourself that it can be helpful to experiment with sitting with aversion. It is not going to kill you.

· Try tuning in to aversion when it is mild, not when it is a ten out of ten. Once you have some experience of feeling what that is like, you can tune in to more intense unpleasant sensations and aversions. Remember that all aspects of our mindfulness practice contribute to our ability to bring mindfulness to sexuality.

THE STRUGGLE: ATTACHMENT FEELS GOOD. WHY WOULD I WANT TO STOP THAT GOOD FEELING?

Just as it is normal to want to move away from unpleasant feelings, it is also normal to want to remain with pleasant feelings.

Strategies

· Practice equanimity by letting go of how tightly you hold on to positive thoughts and feelings.

- Remind yourself that practicing equanimity in your mindfulness does not mean that you have to let go of positive feelings in your life in general.

- Remind yourself that all sensations—positive, negative, or neutral—are impermanent. No matter how much you strive to cling to positive sensations, they will eventually fade away. The good news is that all sensations might come back.

THE STRUGGLE: I COULD TRY ON THE POSITIVE SEXUAL IMAGERY DURING THE EXERCISES IN THE CHAPTER, BUT IT IS TOO HARD TO DO ON MY OWN.

Many women in our past mindfulness groups could follow along with our facilitator's instructions to try on a positive sexual identity, but when they tried doing it at home on their own, they found it impossible.

Strategies

- Start with a positive sexual message that does not feel like too much of a stretch for you, and is about your own experience (not necessarily about your partner's). Perhaps "I like sex" or some version of that.

- Remind yourself that positive statements about yourself can affect how you feel and what you do, even if you do not believe those statements.

- Trust in the science that shows that people who experimentally try on these positive sexual statements respond with stronger sexual arousal than people who do not—even when they do not necessarily believe them!

TIME TO PRACTICE

Before you move on to chapter 8, try the Pleasurable Sensations practice two or more times. Each time, try to use a different sexual tool. For example, you might use a vibrator the first time and watch some erotica the second time. See if you can tune in to the effect on your sensations when you use different sexual tools. When you have completed this exercise, take a few minutes to note the physical sensations and mental sensations (thoughts and emotions) that arose during this exercise and jot them down in your journal along with the date, type of exercise, time, and minutes practiced.

Your informal practice for the week will be the same as the one from chapter 6: to incorporate all five senses into any sexual activity you have with a partner or on your own.

8

Sexual Mindfulness for Two

COUPLES-BASED MINDFULNESS

So far, the mindfulness exercises and other practices in this workbook have been designed so that you can do them on your own. No partner needed! But many of our group participants have said they would like their partner to participate in some of the practices, so this chapter describes three mindfulness exercises you can do with your partner: Back-to-Back Sensing, Mindful Listening, and Sensate Focus.

These exercises work best if both partners are engaged and understand the instructions. Read the instructions together and check in with each other before you start. Can you both set aside other tasks, obligations, and distractions while you do the practice, just as you did when you practiced the earlier exercises alone?

If your partner experiences their own sexual difficulties, they might have negative thoughts about doing any of the following exercises. Reassure them that the exercises are not goal-oriented. They are designed to bring mindfulness to the exercises—no more, no less. If arousal or pleasure occurs for them, these sensations should simply be noticed. They are not to be treated as a trigger for sexual activity. In fact, sensate focus, which I will discuss at length later, works best if sexual activity is completely prohibited.

These exercises also require you to feel safe in your relationship. It is natural to feel a degree of vulnerability when you do this type of exercise, and vulnerability can even be a gateway to fully letting go of anxious thoughts or expectations. However, fear of your partner, extreme worry about their reactions to the exercises, or severe conflict in your relationship may be signs that your relationship requires a different type of help. In that case you might consider consulting with a relationship therapist. If ever you are concerned about your safety, whether by threatened or actual violence, I urge you to reach out for help. The World Health Organization (WHO) has an excellent website on violence against women that you might find helpful (www.who.int/news-room/fact-sheets/detail/violence-against-women).

COMMUNICATION IS KEY

Many people find it challenging to openly communicate their sexual needs to their partner. They may worry that they will hurt a partner's feelings, that it means that they are not "naturally" sexually compatible, or that they or their partner will feel awkward or embarrassed. They may think their partner should already know how to make sex pleasurable for them, even though none of us can read other people's minds.

Here are some general principles of communication recommended by experts in communication and couples therapy. For each suggestion, write down whether you would consider that strategy or what adaptations you would make so that it would work within your own relationship. If you are not in a relationship, you can still imagine how each of the following suggestions, both verbal and nonverbal, might work for you in the future.

VERBAL COMMUNICATION TIPS

· Choose a time when you and your partner are not overly tired or stressed.

- Choose a time when you are feeling calm and able to articulate your need.

- Know what you want—and be honest.

- Use "I" statements rather than "you" statements. When you begin your statements with "I" rather than "you," you focus on your feelings rather than on what you perceive as your partner's flaws. For instance, say "I would love more oral sex—you are so good at it" rather than "You never give me enough oral sex."

- As much as possible, phrase your suggestions in the positive rather than in the negative (e.g., "I love it when you kiss my neck. Could you do that more?"). Sometimes, however, it is important to tell your partner not to do certain things that you dislike.

- Make requests rather than demands.

- Meet your partner halfway. Ask them what they like and listen to their response. Ask what you can do to make their sexual experience better.

- Give your partner time to digest what you say. What you're telling them could be entirely new information to them.

- Revisit your and your partner's sexual needs often to keep the lines of communication open in and out of the bedroom.

NONVERBAL COMMUNICATION TIPS

- Place your hand over your partner's hand and direct it to the right location and indicate the right pressure and speed to bring you pleasure.

- Make noise when you are enjoying what your partner is doing.

- Show your partner how you like to stimulate yourself.

SEXUAL MINDFULNESS FOR TWO

- Smile.

- Make eye contact with your partner.

FORMAL EXERCISE 12:
BACK-TO-BACK SENSING PRACTICE

Back-to-Back Sensing is a mindfulness exercise that involves bringing awareness to the sensations in your body while you are in contact with your partner's body. In addition to noticing the internal sensations in your body, as you did with the Body Scan, you will also bring your attention to the points of contact between your body and your partner's body.

You will be clothed during this practice. If you have a tendency to feel uncomfortably vulnerable during sexual activity, the layers of clothing between your body and your partner's body should reduce the intensity of your vulnerability. If you would like to try it again skin to skin, you can remove layers of clothing on subsequent practices.

WHAT YOU WILL NEED

- Your partner
- Two chairs positioned side by side so that you can sit back to back without the chairback between your bodies, or a comfortable mat that is big enough for you and your partner to sit on back to back
- A quiet space (remember that no space will be totally silent, and that is okay!)
- Comfortable socks or shoes
- Your journal

This will take about fifteen minutes. Your partner will read the instructions to you while you practice mindfulness, and then before proceeding to the Inquiry, you switch roles and you will read the instructions to your partner. There is no audio recording of this practice.

STEP-BY-STEP GUIDE TO BACK-TO-BACK SENSING PRACTICE

The instructions in this practice are given as if you are sitting down with the chair backs beside one another. If you do this exercise standing up back to back, adjust the instructions as required. The partner who is not reading will be invited to close their eyes, but this exercise is about falling awake, not falling asleep, so if you or your partner have a tendency to doze off, keep your eyes open, or open them periodically throughout the meditation.

- Settle into a comfortable sitting position, with your feet flat on the floor. Allow your back to settle against your partner's back in a tall, dignified posture. Allow your eyes to close if this feels comfortable. Open them at any point during the practice and move into a soft, unfocused downward gaze.

- Do your best to stay alert and mentally focused throughout this practice.

- In this exercise, you will become aware of whatever sensations are present in each passing moment and bring an accepting and compassionate attitude toward whatever is arising in your field of awareness, look at it clearly, and see it as it is. It is part of your experience in the moment, for better or for worse. Let go of the tendency, which we all have, to want things to be different from how they are right now, and allow things to be as you find them. Allow yourself to be exactly as you are.

- There is no goal of feeling different or changing what you are experiencing.

- You are not changing your thoughts or becoming more relaxed or less tense. Each of these feelings of tension, restlessness, and doubt can all be observed as sensations that arise, linger, and then move on.

- Whenever some other focus of your attention, such as a physical sensation in another area of the body, a sound, or a thought, becomes predominant, momentarily allow this to be the new focus for your attention and bring the same level of mindful awareness, of acceptance, to that sensation, sound, or thought, continuing to observe it until it is no longer predominant. Then bring your attention back to your breath and to the focus of your attention in that moment.

- Whenever you notice that you have forgotten about the focus of your attention because your attention was engaged in or identifying with the content of a thought, congratulate yourself on becoming aware of that. Notice what your attention had been engaged with and then, with kindness, return your attention to the sensation of your partner's back.

- Gently guide your attention to the sensations of breathing. You are not manipulating your breath in any way, such as trying to make it slower or deeper. You are simply experiencing sensations of breathing as the air moves in and out of your body. Direct your attention to your abdomen and feel the sensations in that region as the breath comes into the body and your belly gently expands and as the breath moves out of your body and your belly deflates.

- Allow your attention to rest on your sensations of breathing moment to moment. Just follow with your mind's eye the rhythmic movements of your belly with each breath.

- Pay attention to the rising of your belly on the in-breath and the falling on the out-breath. Pause there for a few moments.

- Over the next few breaths, gather your attention and move the focus of your attention to the sensations of your partner's back against your own. Allow your attention to rest on what sensations arise for you at this time. There may be sensations of contact, of warmth or coolness, of softness or hardness, of broadness or narrowness.

- Whatever the specific sensations are is not important. Just bring your attention to the sensations of your partner's back against your own. Pause there a while and simply observe what comes up.

- Whenever you notice that your attention has become engaged in or identified with a different sensation, or the content of a thought, just gently acknowledge that this has happened. Bring acceptance and compassion to whatever sensation or thought comes up. Congratulate yourself for noticing that your attention has moved to a different sensation or thought. With that sense of acceptance or compassion, simply guide your attention back to the sensation of your partner's back against your own. Pause there for a few moments.

- When you are ready, expand your field of awareness to include your entire body, from the top of your head to the soles of your feet.

- Pay careful attention to the many individual sensations that arise and pass away within this larger field of awareness, wherever they are located in your body. Allow your attention to move fluidly from sensation to sensation, wherever they arise, momentarily focusing on each one, as it rises and fades in prominence, and, without straining, observe each as clearly as possible. Pause there for a few moments.

- As you come to the end of this practice, perhaps form the intention to bring this moment-to-moment noticing of sensations to the rest of your day. You may want to wiggle your toes and fingers, noticing sensations of movement. You may wish to congratulate yourself on having taken the time and the energy to nourish yourself in this way and to remember that this state of awareness is accessible to you by simply attending to sensations, such as those of the in-breath and the out-breath, in any moment, no matter what is happening, at any time of the day.

- Whenever you're ready, allow your eyes to open if they have been closed.

- Turn around to face your partner and gaze into their eyes for a minute, just observing the shape and color of their eyes.

- Now is the time to pass the instructions to your partner as you switch roles.

- Finally, take a few deep breaths before you move on to the Inquiry.

THE INQUIRY

This Inquiry is an opportunity for you and your partner to share what came up for you during the Back-to-Back Sensing practice. Read the questions and share with one another what you noticed. This is not so much a discussion as a reflection. You can read each question out loud and take turns responding, or you can both share your reflections in a conversation (but do not speak over one another!). Try to spend at least ten minutes with your partner on the following three questions.

QUESTION 1. What did you notice during this practice?

What physical feelings arose for you? What mental sensations arose? What else did you feel? (Remember that partner 1 asks partner 2 and then just listens. Then partner 2 asks partner 1 and then just listens.)

What sensations did you observe? What words would you use to describe the physical sensations? Can you describe those sensations in more detail? Where was the sensation located? Over what area did it extend—how large or small was the sensation? Were you aware of the boundaries of the sensation—where did the sensation end? How intense was the sensation? What were the physical qualities of the sensation (heat, coolness, pinpricks, wavy, etc.)? Did the sensation change over time? How quickly did the sensations come and go or change?

QUESTION 2. How was paying attention to the sensations of contact between your backs different from how you normally notice sensations of contact between your bodies in your day-to-day life?

Have you ever paid attention to your sensations when your backs have been in contact before? What about when other parts of your body are in contact? What made this different from or similar to how you normally pay attention to points of contact between your body and your partner's body?

QUESTION 3. How was this practice relevant to your sexuality?

This is an opportunity to speculate on how this practice of noticing sensations as your backs are in contact might be relevant to your sexuality. There are no right or wrong answers.

Did you observe something about your attention that could be incorporated into sex? Did you learn something about how you pay attention that might be helpful in understanding your difficulties with sex?

END OF THE BACK-TO-BACK SENSING PRACTICE

Congratulations to you and your partner for doing this exercise. Many couples I have worked with who do it state that they usually do not pay that much attention to the feelings of their body coming into contact with their partner's body. Many also state that the strict instruction to remain in the moment was a different way of being with their partner's body, as they would often be triggered into thinking about sex if they touched their partner's body for that long. They also described feeling new sensations that they were previously unaware of, both within their own body and at the points of contact with their partner's body.

What kinds of thoughts came up for you during this practice? Were there any worries? Anxieties? Any anticipation of negative outcomes? Sexual pleasure? A desire to touch more? Write your answers in your journal.

This mindfulness exercise is a good introduction to a more intimate mindful touching exercise you'll do with your partner later in this chapter called Sensate Focus. But first, we will practice a partnered mindfulness exercise that involves not touch but listening.

FORMAL EXERCISE 13:
MINDFUL LISTENING PRACTICE

During the Mindfulness of Thoughts practice in chapter 4 I invited you to pay attention to sounds—both inside and outside the room. In that practice, I guided you to bring your attention to the qualities of sound reaching your ears, such as pitch, tone, and volume. This practice also involves sounds, but this time, instead of just receiving sounds, you will practice really paying attention while listening. You and your partner will take turns talking and listening mindfully. By using mindfulness skills in this way, you will practice what is most likely a very different way of communicating with one another.

WHAT YOU WILL NEED

Take a moment to decide who will talk first. This will be Person A. Person B will listen first.

- A quiet space (remember that no space will be totally silent, and that is okay!)
- A timer or stopwatch
- Two chairs

This practice will take about fifteen minutes. There is no audio recording of this practice. The first part of the exercise will last for five minutes. Have your stopwatch or timer ready to use. As this mindfulness practice is different from all of the previous individual mindfulness practices done in this workbook, you may wish to read through the instructions below first before attempting it with your partner.

STEP-BY-STEP GUIDE TO MINDFUL LISTENING

- Person A begins by sharing their current experience and Person B is to listen without talking—noticing thoughts, sensing emotions, and sensations in their body as they do so.

- During this exercise, both Person A and Person B simply notice physical sensations, thoughts, and sounds or smells in their environment.

- During this first part of the exercise, Person A shares whatever sensations they are noticing in this moment. These may be sensations in the body, in the environment, or in the mind. Describe those sensations in detail, without labeling them.

- Use the language of bare sensations to describe any bodily sensations.

- For mental sensations, or thoughts, you might say "I am having memory thoughts" or "I am having planning thoughts" or even "I am having catastrophic thoughts" without going into the specifics of what each thought is.

- Person B is to listen mindfully and may notice reactions to Person A or perhaps reactions within themselves but does not say anything.

- Each person is intentionally bringing awareness to their own experience in the moment, and also noticing changes in their experience from moment to moment.

- There may be silences, and this is normal. Do not move into a conversation but notice the temptation to do so, should this arise.

- Sit with the silence until a sensation arises that you wish to share.

- After five minutes have elapsed, Person B can reflect on what they heard.

- Set your timer or stopwatch for two minutes.

- Person B then briefly shares their experience of just listening to Person A. If Person B has a question about what Person A was saying or communicating, they can ask at this time.

- Remember that this is not a conversation but an opportunity for Person B to show curiosity about Person A's experience. Person A should listen mindfully to Person B and then answer the question as best they can.

- If silence occurs, simply sit with it. It does not mean anything is wrong.

- After two minutes, stop and switch roles.

- Set your stopwatch or timer for five minutes and repeat the steps above, with Person B sharing what they are experiencing.

- After you have both been both speaker and listener, you can move on to the Inquiry.

THE INQUIRY

This Inquiry is an opportunity for you and your partner to share what came up for you during the mindful listening exercise. As you did with the Back-to-Back Sensing practice, reflect on your sensations—both in your body and in your mind. This is not so much a discussion as it is a reflection. Try to spend at least ten minutes on the following three questions with your partner. Each of you can answer question 1 before proceeding to question 2, and so on.

QUESTION 1. What did you notice during this exercise?

What physical sensations arose for you? What mental sensations arose? What else did you feel?

As a reminder, Person A reflects on what sensations they noticed while Person B just listens without speaking. What does it feel like to just be with the silences?

QUESTION 2. How was mindful listening to your partner in this way different from how you might normally listen to them while they are speaking?

You and your partner can have a free-flowing discussion in response to this question. Try to really focus on what felt different in this practice compared to how you normally speak and listen to one another in your life.

Did you notice an urge to talk while your partner was listening? What happened to that urge? As you were speaking to your partner, how was talking in this way different from how you talk to them in your day-to-day life?

QUESTION 3. How might this mindful listening exercise be relevant to your sexuality? How might this way of communication be relevant to your intimacy?

It is fine to go out on a limb here and speculate on how your observations in this practice may be relevant to your sexual response or sexual encounters with one another. Remember that there is no right or wrong answer. This question is about contemplating in what ways mindfulness might be useful in your sexual relationship.

Write your reflections in your journal.

END OF THE MINDFUL LISTENING PRACTICE

Congratulations to you and your partner for taking part in this mindful listening practice. It may have felt strange to have experienced that much silence together. Many of us become impatient with silence and feel that we need to fill it. In this exercise, the silence is an opportunity to observe in more depth what sensations are there when you truly just listen. Sometimes the silences can be transformational! Sometimes silence can allow a person to reflect more deeply on what they are feeling, and this can be an opportunity for the listener to learn something new about their partner.

When we have done this mindful listening exercise with couples in our research program, many of them say that they have never, even after decades in their relationship, just listened to what their partner was saying. During the Inquiry, partners often state that when they were in the role of speaker and just tuning in to their experience and describing it, without the goal of changing anything, they felt that they did not censor what they were saying. This feels very powerful for many people in relationships, especially those who say they feel they can't speak without fear of being judged.

This exercise may bring up a number of different sensations for you, some of which may be familiar to you now, while others will be new. Some observations that may come up include:

- the experience of connection
- mindfulness during communication
- a sense of self in relation to another
- the kindness of just listening
- noticing needs—for example, the need for reassurance
- noticing discomfort
- noticing your own needs versus the needs of your partner

Mindful listening is important because communication and listening are core to satisfying sex. Just as communicating about your preferences, likes, dislikes, and distress regarding sex in an open, honest way can be key to receiving touch and stimulation that feel right for you, listening mindfully will allow you to respond to your partner in a nonreactive and nonjudgmental way. It also puts you directly in touch with how you are feeling when your partner speaks and buys time to allow you to pause, reflect, and then act instead of offering a knee-jerk reflexive response.

Mindful listening and mindful speaking are important tools in the next mindfulness exercise: Sensate Focus. This is my favorite couples-based mindfulness exercise, and it is also a favorite among many of the participants in our mindful sex programs.

SENSATE FOCUS: A MINDFULNESS EXERCISE IN DISGUISE

William Masters and Virginia Johnson have been described by many in the field of sex therapy and research as the father and mother of modern-day sex therapy. They sought to understand the nature of human sexual response, and they did so by using a variety of psychophysiological tools (e.g., electromyography to measure muscle tone) to measure different aspects of sexual response as people became aroused and engaged in sexual activity in a research setting, with the two researchers often watching just steps away. They drew on the results of their research to develop the first model of sexual response.

In making new discoveries about factors that facilitate sexual arousal, they also observed factors that contribute to sexual problems—most notably, *spectatoring*. Spectatoring is when a person focuses on themselves from a third-person point of view during sexual activity instead of focusing on their partner and the sex they are having. It is as if you are watching yourself from a distance and are not connected to yourself in the moment. They posited that spectatoring can increase performance anxiety and therefore interfere with sexual arousal.

Masters and Johnson developed sensate focus therapy as an antidote to spectatoring. They reasoned that sensate focus could reduce spectatoring and the associated performance anxiety simply by teaching partners to be in the present moment and let go of any goals of experiencing arousal and orgasm. Johnson led the development of sensate focus by drawing on her experience as a young child when her mother would soothe her in times of emotional turmoil through touch. Sensate focus involves systematic touching between partners, with the goal of reducing anxiety and worries about sex. It does not have the goal of triggering sexual arousal.

Masters and Johnson tracked the outcomes from their sensate focus program, which at the time involved in-patient treatment for two to three weeks while couples stayed in a hotel, away from their homes, families, and obligations, and dedicated much of their time each day to practicing sensate focus and seeing Masters and Johnson for sex therapy. Masters and Johnson's research showed that their program was remarkably effective in both the short and long term. When participants were assessed five years after completing the program, most had maintained the improvements they had made during the program.

Traditional Masters and Johnson sensate focus therapy has been criticized because it is unrealistic for many (in fact, probably most) couples to get away to a hotel for two to three weeks. Today, sex therapists prescribe a modified, more accessible version of sensate focus. Although Masters and Johnson never used the terminology of mindfulness as they described the steps of sensate focus, it is evident that mindfulness is at the heart of the exercises: couples are taught to pay attention to each sensation, nonjudgmentally and without acting on it, and just observing the sensations as they are.

The goal of sensate focus is to teach couples to remain in the present moment and focused on the sensations that arise while receiving intimate touch from a partner, without focusing on or anticipating sexual arousal or orgasm. While a partner is giving touch, they too have an opportunity to notice what sensations are coming up in their own body. It has three stages: Stage 1 involves touching everywhere except the chest/breast and genitals, Stage 2 includes those areas during touching, and Stage 3 involves mutual touching all over plus penetration (if applicable). As the couple progresses through the three stages, they each try to remain as mindful as possible and to observe but not become consumed by any negative thoughts that emerge and instead redirect their attention to touch sensations. In all three stages, the couple is asked to not engage in sexual activity immediately afterwards.

SEXUAL MINDFULNESS FOR TWO

To my mind, there are three main goals of sensate focus:

1. **Relaxation.** Truly relaxing while receiving touch from your partner can reduce your feelings of anxiety and calm an activated stress response system, and so maximize the likelihood of arousal, pleasure, and enjoyment.

2. **Mindfulness.** Sensate focus gives you the opportunity to fully tune in to the experience of contact with your partner, including physical sensations (pressure, temperature, texture) and mental sensations (thoughts, expectations, memories). You can practice taking the attitude that whatever happens, happens. And you can tune in to touch nonjudgmentally, moment by moment.

3. **Sexual communication.** Since the receiver is providing feedback to the giver of touch ("Keep touching there," "That feels good," "That is too hard," "Move to the right a bit"), this is really good sexual communication practice that you can take into sexual encounters in the future.

FORMAL EXERCISE 14: SENSATE FOCUS PRACTICE

Planning is essential in sensate focus, but it does not have to be clinical, dry, or boring, as some people may believe. When participants balk at the mention of planning, I ask them what else they do in their life that is meaningful, valued, and fun and involves at least one other person that is not planned? The response is inevitably "Nothing!" When you plan for this exercise, you increase the likelihood that you'll have privacy, that your head and heart will be in a good place, and that each of you shows up on time!

Another way to prepare yourself for Sensate Focus is to tell yourself that you will be open to receiving feedback. When you are touching your partner (being the *giver*), they will be providing gentle feedback to you about what that touching feels like and perhaps also a request to touch them in a different way (being the *receiver*). Guiding each other during sensate focus is a crucial part of the exercise, and it will help you develop—or rediscover—a happy, healthy sexual life together. You cannot read your partner's mind about their precise likes and dislikes when it comes to touch (and sex), no matter how long you have been together. It is "safer" to assume that you know nothing about how your partner likes to be touched rather than thinking you know what their preferences are and being wrong. With practice, you will feel much more comfortable giving this kind of feedback to your partner (and receiving it).

A final way you can get ready for sensate focus is by continuing to do your daily mindfulness practice. Since sensate focus is really mindfulness but with a partner (and no clothes!), the same skills of present-moment, nonjudgmental awareness that you have been cultivating over these past several weeks will come in handy for this exercise.

WHAT YOU WILL NEED

· Your partner
· A bed
· A quiet space (remember that no space will be totally silent, and that is okay!)
· A timer or stopwatch
· All distractions removed
· A lock on the door (if you are concerned about someone walking in)
· A comfortable room temperature (neither too hot nor too cold)

STEP-BY-STEP GUIDE TO SENSATE FOCUS: STAGE 1

- Set your timer for 15 minutes.

- Take off all your clothes, if you feel comfortable, and lie on the bed facing one another. If one or both of you feels uncomfortable, you can do the first few sensate focus practices in your underwear.

- Designate the giver and the receiver.

- The giver touches the receiver according to the giver's own curiosity about where to touch, without any set "agenda." The breasts/chest and genitals are off limits for this stage. The receiver can also choose other areas that they don't want to be touched during this stage.

- The giver takes note of the temperature, pressure, and texture at their fingertips while touching.

- The receiver focuses on these same qualities of touch in the location where they are being touched. Here is where your mindfulness skills of tuning in to touch, temperature, vibration, texture, roughness or smoothness, intensity, precise location, and other qualities of the touch come in handy.

- The receiver can provide some gentle nonverbal feedback to the giver of the touch if the touch feels very unpleasant, such as ticklish (by moving or applying pressure to the giver's hand).

- The receiver can also provide gentle verbal feedback such as "Move to the left" or "A bit softer please."

- The giver should feel free to touch all parts of the receiver's body (except the breasts/chest, genitals, and any other areas of the body that the receiver has asked not to be touched). Oral sex and any form of penetration are also off limits.

- Once 15 minutes have elapsed, the giver of the touch becomes the receiver, and the receiver becomes the giver.

- Follow the steps above.

- After 15 minutes, relax together for a few minutes without touching one another.

THE INQUIRY

Take a few moments to mindfully ask your partner what the experience, as both giver and receiver, was like. Listen with awareness and without interrupting. Take note of what sensations come up for you as your partner shares what they observed during the exercise. Try to spend about fifteen minutes on this Inquiry before moving on to your next activity, or before going to sleep. Avoid sexual activity immediately after Sensate Focus, or the next time that you practice it you might find yourself anticipating sex instead of immersing yourself in the exercise.

Many couples do about five to ten Stage 1 Sensate Focus practices before proceeding to Stage 2. Both participants need to be undressed during Stage 2 because it involves genital touch. If either of you feels uncomfortable being naked, work through this discomfort in Stage 1 before you move on. This might take a few weeks or a few months. Take as much time as you need. When you are ready, follow the instructions below.

STEP-BY-STEP GUIDE TO SENSATE FOCUS: STAGE 2

- Set your timer for 15 minutes.

- Take all of your clothes off and lie on your bed facing one another.

- As in Stage 1, you will designate a giver and a receiver of touch.

- This time, the giver will touch all parts of the body, including the breasts/chest, genitals, and any areas that were avoided in Stage 1. Oral sex and any form of penetration are still off limits.

- The giver is still touching according to their own curiosity rather than to provide pleasure to the receiver, and is trying to set aside their beliefs and conceptions of how and where the receiver likes to be touched and instead trying to touch all over equally. They continue to notice their own sensations as they are delivering touch.

- Continue in this way for 15 minutes.

- After 15 minutes, switch roles so that the giver is now the receiver, and vice versa.

- After 15 minutes, stop the touching and relax together for a few minutes without touching one another.

THE INQUIRY

Ask your partner what it was like to receive touch in the erogenous parts of their body. Could they focus on the sensations themselves? What thoughts/mental sensations arose for them? Did they experience arousal? If so, what did they do with the arousal?

Sometimes specific thoughts and fears can arise, such as "What if I don't get aroused while my partner is touching me?" These types of mental events are far from unusual. When you recognize these thoughts and "let them be," they lose their power and can dissipate on their own. Since sensate focus is non-goal-oriented, you and your partner are not trying to get anywhere during or after the practice. The goal is simply to observe all that arises, just as it is.

STEP-BY-STEP GUIDE TO SENSATE FOCUS: STAGE 3

- Take off all of your clothes and lie on your bed facing one another.

- Start by giving your partner non-genital and non-breast/chest touching followed by breast/chest and genital touching.

- Then your partner will do the same to you.

- After that, you will progress to mutual touching of each other. Each person continues to touch according to their own curiosity and to focus on their own physical sensations. Oral sex and intercourse are still off limits.

- During this stage you will progress to rubbing your genitals against each other. You may feel ready to do this the first time you practice Stage 3, or you may want to do Stage 3 a few times without genitals touching one another first.

- If your partner is male, get on top of him and use his penis to touch your own genitals mindfully and without rushing. Once he has achieved an erection, you can insert his penis inside your vagina (or anus), without initiating thrusting and while remaining very mindful of all sensations.

- If your partner is female, get on top of her and slowly rub your clitoris and vulva against hers mindfully and without rushing.

- Don't worry about your or your partner's level of pleasure. Set aside any expectations you have.

- You each touch one another's body at the same time and focus on sensations arising for you.

- Continue to do this entire exercise for fifteen to thirty minutes.

- Once you stop, discuss what that was like.

THE INQUIRY

Ask your partner what it was like to engage in mutual touch where you were simultaneously noticing sensations in your own body and the points of contact with your partner's body. What effect did a slow penetration or slow rubbing have on you? Did you resist the urge to thrust or initiate? What was the quality of your sensations? How long did they linger? What thoughts/mental sensations arose for you? Were you aroused? If so, what did you do with the arousal? Take turns to answer these questions.

END OF THE SENSATE FOCUS PRACTICE

Sensate Focus is an advanced exercise that you may wish to consider trying with the guidance of a counselor/therapist who can answer any questions and troubleshoot any difficulties. It is not just for individuals and couples who have sexual difficulties. It can also be helpful for couples who want to introduce more mindfulness into their already satisfying sex life.

EDUCATION ABOUT SEX: REASONS FOR SEX

People have many reasons for having sex, and they need not be in response to feeling sexual desire. In 2007, researchers Cindy Meston and David Buss at the University of Texas at Austin asked three thousand men and women about their reasons for having sex and found approximately 237 reasons!

Many of the reasons concerned the pleasure, arousal, and enjoyment the participants anticipated deriving from the sexual activity. Even if at the moment of deciding to initiate sex or accept a partner's invitation they did not feel any strong sexual urge or drive, they said that they expected to feel some desire a bit later in the encounter once they got "into it." Many spoke of feeling closer to their partners by being sexual; of wanting to show love, affection, commitment, and attraction to their partner; and also wanting to feel better about themselves—more attractive, accepted, and "normal."

As we noted earlier, sometimes people's reasons for having sex can be negative, such as to avoid a fight with a partner or to mitigate conflict in their relationship. We call these *avoidance-related motives* since they are designed to avoid something negative. If a person exclusively has sex for avoidance-related reasons, resentment can build over time. In contrast, *approach-related reasons* are what we would consider positive reasons—for example, wanting to achieve emotional intimacy or connection.

A person in a sexually neutral state who has approach-related (= good) reasons to be sexual, such as wanting to be closer to their partner, may require a sexual stimulus to generate sexual arousal. That sexual stimulus needs to be processed by the brain in order to elicit the sensations and emotions that we call sexual arousal. A consideration of the context or environment can be complex. It includes the interpersonal context (the physical space around you, privacy, safety, how you feel about your partner, and whether what they are doing is "turning you on or off").

Now might be a good time for you to review the sexual response cycle you learned about in chapter 3, which prioritizes responsive sexual desire over spontaneous sexual desire. Since this current chapter is focused on exercises you can do with your partner, try to read over the list of reasons for sex below together. Note that this list is only a snapshot compared with the list the University of Texas at Austin researchers compiled! In reading through the list together, you can discuss how compelling you find each reason as a motive to engage in sex or not. Or you could each have a hard copy of the list and separately check off the reasons that resonate with you. Then swap your lists and discuss your choices. You might both be surprised.

- I desired emotional closeness (i.e., intimacy).
- I felt insecure.
- I hadn't had sex for a while.
- I realized I was in love.
- I saw my partner naked and could not resist.
- I thought it would help me to fall asleep.
- I thought it would relax me.
- I wanted my partner to notice me.
- I wanted the adventure/excitement.
- I wanted my partner to feel good about themselves.
- I wanted the pure pleasure.
- I wanted to experience an orgasm.
- I wanted to act out a fantasy.
- I wanted to burn calories.
- I wanted to celebrate a birthday or anniversary or special occasion.
- I wanted to communicate at a "deeper" level.
- I wanted to experience the physical pleasure of sex.
- I wanted to express my love for my partner.
- I wanted to feel attractive.
- I wanted to feel powerful.
- I wanted to get a favor from my partner.
- I wanted to get out of doing something.
- I wanted to get rid of a headache.
- I wanted to get the most out of life.
- I wanted to have a child.
- I wanted to improve my sexual skills.
- I wanted to intensify my relationship.
- I wanted to keep warm.
- I wanted to lift my partner's spirits.
- I wanted to release anxiety/stress.
- I wanted to say "Goodbye."

- I wanted to say "I'm sorry."
- I wanted to say "I've missed you."
- I wanted to say "Thank you."
- I wanted to see what all the fuss is about.
- I wanted to show my affection to my partner.
- I wanted to welcome my partner home.
- I was "horny."
- I was bored.
- I was frustrated and needed relief.
- It seemed like the natural next step in my relationship.
- It would allow me to "get sex out of my system" so that I could focus on other things.
- It's exciting, adventurous.
- My partner had a desirable body.
- My partner had done something nice for me.
- My partner was too "hot" (sexy) to resist.

STRUGGLES AND STRATEGIES

The struggles below relate to the communication practices as well as the three partnered mindfulness practices in this chapter: Back-to-Back Sensing, Mindful Listening, and Sensate Focus. As always, the strategies are meant as a guide, and I encourage you to come up with your own. You could also have a conversation with your partner if any of these or other struggles arise and try to brainstorm solutions together.

THE STRUGGLE: COMMUNICATING WITH "I" LANGUAGE IS CHALLENGING.

When you feel angry, resentful, irritated, or sad because you believe your partner did something wrong, you might automatically tell them what they did wrong. After all, it was their action (or inaction) that led you to feel this way, right? Even if your partner is responsible for what happened, pointing a finger at them will put them on the defensive and possibly prevent an amicable resolution of the issue.

Strategies

· Rehearse how you will express your issue (or request) using "I" language. You may need to practice saying this out loud to yourself a few times.

· Remind yourself you are using "I" language because it centers the conversation on your feelings rather than on your partner's flaws.

· Remind yourself that with practice and intention, even old, familiar patterns of communication can change.

THE STRUGGLE: PAUSING TO LISTEN WHILE MY PARTNER SPEAKS IS REALLY HARD.

The reality is that people in a long-term relationship may think they know what their partner is thinking before they even say it. This makes pausing, listening, and being silent challenging. If you think you know what your partner is going to say, why wait in silence?

Strategies

· Remind yourself that mind-reading is only a fallacy. There is no evidence that the longer you are in a relationship, the more accurate you are at reading your partner's mind.

· Open and honest communication about sex is found to be a predictor of long-term sexual satisfaction. Part of healthy sexual communication is the ability to listen.

· Count to ten (or twenty) while your partner is speaking to ensure that you do not cut them off.

THE STRUGGLE: I WORRY THAT IF I PROVIDE VERBAL FEED-
BACK TO MY PARTNER ABOUT HOW TO TOUCH ME THEY WILL
BE OFFENDED.

Many people do not give feedback about how to improve sexual
stimulation for fear their partner will be upset. As a result, they
may spend years (or even decades) receiving inadequate or even
painful touch.

Strategies

· Accepting that you cannot read your partner's mind and that
they cannot read yours can free up the guilt you may feel about
giving your partner feedback about how they are touching you.

· When you are providing constructive feedback to your partner
about their touch, fold it into positive feedback about something
else that you really like about how they touch you.

· Choose your timing carefully. Do not provide this kind of feedback during a disagreement. Wait until you are both feeling
good or relaxed.

THE STRUGGLE: I DON'T THINK MY PARTNER WILL WANT TO
DO ANY OF THE COUPLES-BASED MINDFULNESS EXERCISES
WITH ME.

Whether you are assuming that your partner will not do the
couples-based mindfulness exercises or your partner told you
that they would not, this can be a frustrating situation—especially since these exercises work, and you have nothing to lose
by trying!

Strategies

· The exercises are likely new to you and to your partner. You had
to muster up the motivation to do them, and your partner might
have to do the same. Offer gentle encouragement to them to
help them see the value in doing the exercise with you.

SEXUAL MINDFULNESS FOR TWO

- You could try sharing some of the science supporting these exercises. You could also mention now and again the possibility of trying them and build up to the "ask."

THE STRUGGLE: AFTER WE PRACTICE SENSATE FOCUS, WE WANT TO HAVE SEX, BUT YOU HAVE SAID IT IS NOT PERMITTED.

Traditional sensate focus programs forbid any kind of sexual activity for the weeks in which people are working on the exercises. However, contemporary sensate focus programs simply instruct couples to not engage in sex right after their practice, but say it is fine to schedule it for other times.

Strategies

- Plan sex! And plan it for times outside of the days that you are practicing sensate focus.

- Remind yourself that removing sex from your relationship equation allows you and your partner to fully immerse yourself in the Sensate Focus exercise without worrying about whether sex will happen and potentially facing performance-related concerns.

TIME TO PRACTICE

Before you move on to the last chapter, try to practice the verbal and nonverbal communication strategies in this chapter at least once a day. If you have time, you could do one of the couples-based mindfulness exercises every second day. Practice the Sensate Focus exercise once a week. Your informal mindfulness practice will be to bring more mindful awareness to all (sexual and nonsexual) interactions with your partner.

9

What about Me? Mindful Sex for Other Populations

CULTIVATING SEXUAL DESIRE THROUGH MINDFULNESS IS NOT JUST FOR WOMEN

This chapter covers a range of other topics related to mindful sex that a variety of people have asked me about—especially after *Better Sex through Mindfulness* was published, when I received many emails from readers asking whether the book and the science of mindfulness were only applicable to women. Most of my research has focused on applying mindfulness to improve the lives of women, including gynecologic cancer survivors, women with a history of sexual abuse, women seeking treatment for low desire, and women with Provoked Vestibulodynia, as well as others, which is why my first book focused on women's sexual health.

However, mindfulness is most definitely for everyone. This chapter therefore focuses on mindful sex for men, gender-diverse individuals, and people wishing to use mindfulness alongside their sexual response enhancing medications. If you do not identify as a woman, I still encourage you to read through chapters 1 to 8, as I will be referring to them and the practices described in them in this chapter.

MINDFUL SEX FOR MEN

When *Better Sex through Mindfulness* was published I received countless emails from men who had read it and were successfully applying the principles of mindfulness I explain in it to their own sex lives. They wondered why *Better Sex through Mindfulness* was written only for women, given that men also experience performance anxiety, stress, low sexual desire, worrisome thoughts, lack of confidence, distractions, and catastrophizing thoughts that interfere with their sexual function. Could the mindfulness exercises I had written for women be adapted for men to use?

In a word: yes. All of the mindfulness exercises that I discuss in the context of women's sexuality can be used by men. The rationale for why mindfulness can benefit women's sexuality also applies to how it can benefit men's sexuality. *Better Sex through Mindfulness* is for everybody—as is the workbook you are holding in your hands.

In the past few years, my research team and our colleagues in a sexual medicine center in Vancouver, British Columbia, have evaluated the effects of mindfulness-based groups for men with sexual concerns—specifically, men with situational erectile dysfunction who have no difficulties achieving erection when they are engaging in solo sexual activity but who lose their erections, or cannot achieve one at all, when they are with a partner. We recruited men whose situational erectile dysfunction was due to psychological factors, such as fear of performance failure, general anxiety, worries, or distractions. Four weeks of mindfulness training led to significantly improved sexual functioning and sexual satisfaction, and the men in the program reported an increased ability to observe their own experiences without judgment. As a result of our research, many clinics now offer mindfulness as a first-line treatment for men with similar sexual concerns.

My research team has also administered mindfulness in a group format to survivors of prostate cancer and their partners. Groups consisting of four couples, on average, took part in four sessions, each two weeks apart, focused on mindfulness skills and sex education. The program led to moderate improvements in the participating couples' sexual satisfaction and large improvements in their ability to be mindful. Interviews at the end of mindfulness treatment with survivors and their partners revealed that their participation in the groups led them to view prostate cancer as a couple's disease and that the group format was a key part of the therapeutic effects of mindfulness. Most of the men who participated in the groups had permanent erection problems, leaving them frustrated both with their health-care providers and with the oral medications that were not restoring their erections as the men had hoped. However, mindfulness offered them an opportunity to explore other ways of being sexual, in a non-judgmental way. As they experimented with other kinds of sexual activity outside of intercourse, and used their mindful awareness skills to tune in to these sensations, their distress significantly decreased and their enjoyment of sexual activities increased.

I routinely use mindfulness with men who are struggling with low sexual desire too. In the same way that doing the Body Scan, 3-Minute Breathing Space, and Mindfulness of Thoughts practices over time helps women tune in to their own feelings of sexual arousal and let distracting or judgmental thoughts pass by like a running stream, mindfulness helps cultivate sexual desire in men.

MINDFUL SEX FOR GENDER-DIVERSE FOLKS

What about people who are on the beautiful rainbow spectrum of gender identity? Trans, nonbinary, agender, gender queer, and gender fluid people comprise up to 2 percent of the population. Although the rates of sexual concerns among these populations are unknown, we do know that these folks can also experience struggles with low desire, lack of sexual arousal, difficulties with orgasm, pain with sex, sexual dissatisfaction, and distress associated with sexual activity and that mindfulness can be helpful to them.

Over the years, a number of gender-diverse people have participated in our mindfulness-based groups of women, and they have benefited in the same way that cis-gender women have. They have shared with me that they appreciate having an opportunity to benefit from the same sex therapy and mindful sex skills that women have access to, in particular because there are well-known systemic barriers that prevent gender-diverse people from accessing health-care services. Some gender-diverse participants have also shared with me that the mindfulness skills they acquired in group programs have helped them with other areas of their lives in which they face anxiety, discrimination, or stereotyping. They also report to me a sense of validation that their sexual concerns are real and that there are tools available to help them cultivate desire and arousal. In my view, the tools and therapies available for addressing sexual health concerns should be equally accessible and available to everyone.

The Body Scan introduced in chapter 2 refers to anatomical parts of the body that correspond with those assigned female at birth. A gender-neutral Body Scan can be found on my website (loribrotto.com).

HOW CAN MINDFULNESS BE COMBINED WITH MEDICATIONS TO BOOST SEXUALITY IN PEOPLE WITH ERECTION DIFFICULTIES?

A number of medications have been approved in countries around the world to treat erection difficulties, including Viagra (sildenafil), Levitra (vardenafil), and Cialis (tadalafil). These medications block the natural mechanisms that turn off sexual arousal, and thus allow sexual arousal to continue. Specifically, the body naturally releases nitric oxide, which then activates a chain of chemical reactions that culminate in the muscles in the penis relaxing, more blood flowing in, and an erection being the end result.

These erection-promoting medications block phosphodiesterase type-5 (PDE5), an enzyme that blocks the cascade of reactions that leads to erection, and essentially make it easier for an erection to occur and to last. In other words, these medications still rely on triggers for sexual arousal to take place, but once the arousal pathway has started, the medications facilitate erection by blocking the erection inhibitors.

Here is where mindfulness comes in. Because mindfulness can assist you in tuning in to sexual triggers, paying attention to the early signs of arousal, letting distractions and other self-judgments go, and otherwise promoting a state of attention to sexual signals, it pairs nicely with these medications. These drugs cannot act on their own, as they do nothing to alter attention to sexual stimuli or reduce negative self-talk. Mindfulness is the critical first step to start the sexual response engine, and then these medications kick in to promote continuing arousal.

My colleagues at the BC Centre for Sexual Medicine in Vancouver routinely combine mindfulness with erection-promoting medications. In fact, this combination has become their standard mode of therapy. If you have been prescribed one of these medications, try adopting a mindfulness practice and doing the Body Scan before taking your pill. I'd love to hear how it works for you!

COMBINING MINDFULNESS WITH PRO-ERECTION MEDICATIONS PRACTICE

This brief mindfulness practice starts when you take your pro-erection medication. It takes elements of the Body Scan, the

Breathing Space, and the Mindfulness of Thoughts meditation, and refers to "The Guest House," the poem in chapter 7. You'll be engaging in mindfulness on your own first, then eliciting a sexual fantasy, and then transitioning into sexual activity with your partner in a planned encounter. After you have ingested your medication, follow the instructions below.

- Get into a comfortable position on your chair or in your bed.

- Take a moment to tune in to your body and pay attention to any feelings that arise now that you have taken your medication.

- There may also be thoughts. Note any emotional quality to these thoughts and try as best as you can to observe them from a distance without being consumed by them.

- Ask yourself if you are feeling anticipation. If you are, where do you sense this in your body? Can you tune in to the details of what makes up that anticipation? Where is it located and how intense is it? Can you draw the boundaries around the different sensations and feelings you have?

- Spend a few minutes tuning in to your breathing. Where do you feel the breath sensations? At your belly? At your chest? At your nostrils?

- Try to remain with your breath sensations even if thoughts are trying to capture your attention. If the thoughts become more intense, you can make them the focus of your attention for a few minutes. Try to note the type of thought that is arising. Is it a planning thought? A memory thought? An emotional thought? Without getting wrapped up in the content of the thought, try to observe its qualities and also what sensations are arising in your body as you take note of the thought.

- If the imagery of sitting on the bank of a stream, with the stream representing your thoughts, is helpful, you can evoke that image now. You can also use any other imagery that is helpful for keeping these mental events "at a distance."

- If you like, you can evoke a sexual image in your mind. This could be one that is exciting to you and stimulates you. Try to engage all of your senses to make that sexual fantasy come alive for you.

- After a few minutes of evoking the fantasy, take note of the sensations in your body. Move your attention down to your genital area and see if you can detect any intensity there. Where do you feel sensations? What do they feel like?

- If you had planned to engage in sexual activity with a partner, you might choose this moment to transition to that activity in whatever way feels natural for you, and acceptable in your relationship.

- Carry this mindful self-awareness with you as you begin to touch, stimulate, and engage sexually with your partner.

- When mental events start to dominate, treat them as "guests" at the door. You can invite them in with the same acceptance and openness as you show toward invited guests.

- Throughout the sexual encounter, try to keep your focus on your physical sensations, as well as the points of contact between you and your partner.

- In your journal, write down your observations from this practice. In addition, think about how using mindfulness along with your medication provided a different experience from when you have relied on medication alone.

You can modify the instructions above in any way that better suits the particulars of your situation and environment. The intention of this practice is for you to invoke mindful awareness and use it to pay attention to any emerging sensations after you've taken your medication and then to retain that mindful self-awareness as you engage in sexual activity. Mindfulness is needed to elicit arousal, and the medication is needed to retain it. They work in concert with one another.

What about medications for women's sexual health concerns? Some countries have approved medications for low sexual desire in women, including Addyi (flibanserin) and Vyleesi (bremelanotide), both of which have been approved by the Food and Drug Administration (USA) and Health Canada. These medications act differently. Flibanserin affects neurochemicals in the brain called norepinephrine, dopamine, and serotonin, and it must be consumed daily for at least eight weeks before it starts to work. Bremelanotide affects the melanocortin system in the brain and should be consumed only when needed. (The melanocortin system is associated with regulation of food intake and metabolism.) Although mindfulness has never been tested in conjunction with these medications, given the scientifically supported evidence of mindfulness for low desire and sexual response, I imagine that it could bolster their effects.

MINDFUL SEX IS FOR EVERYONE

I see no limits to how mindfulness can be applied to many aspects of sexuality in the lives of everybody. My hope is for continued investment in research on these different applications of mindfulness discussed above, so that there is science to support the practice. In the meantime, I encourage you to share the information you've learned, and the skills you've practiced here, with another person you think might benefit from this mindfulness approach to sexuality. After all, mindful sex is for everyone.

Acknowledgments

THIS WORKBOOK IS in direct response to the numerous requests I received after the publication of *Better Sex through Mindfulness*. Clinicians wanted a different approach to address their patients' sexual health issues than treatment as usual or hearing about their clients resorting to experimental, unscientific, and often expensive remedies. And many people experiencing sexual difficulties reached out to me having become intrigued by mindfulness and now they wanted the "how to" guide. This urging from clinicians and treatment-seekers combined with the impetus provided by the incredibly brilliant team at Greystone Books (Rob Sanders) was the nudge I needed to take the contents of our in-person mindful sex groups and create this workbook. I'm thankful for the excellent team of editors (Nancy Flight, Lesley Cameron, and others) who ensured clarity in the mindful sex exercises you'll see in this workbook.

Given that the mindful sex approach described in this workbook has been the subject of my research over the past twenty years, I am especially grateful to the funding agencies, my university department of Obstetrics and Gynaecology, and the University of British Columbia for providing the space, support, and infrastructure to carry out the science while running these mindful sex groups.

I am also indebted to the team of students, collaborators, and colleagues who have been a part of this scientific endeavor with me since 2002. Without a doubt, gratitude needs to be extended to the many thousands of people who have participated in our groups and with curiosity and openness (sometimes along with healthy skepticism) were willing to take a chance on eight weeks of compassionate awareness training applied to their own sex lives. Their feedback and experiences over the years have directly contributed to this program.

I wish to thank my career-long collaborator and friend, Dr. Rosemary Basson, who retired in 2021 after an impactful career as a premier teacher of sexual medicine at the University of British Columbia. Dr. Basson has been a longstanding co-investigator in my research, and a contributor to the original mindful sex treatment manual that influenced this workbook. Though she has stepped away formally from teaching sexual medicine and seeing individuals with sexual health concerns, her influence continues through the many hundreds of trainees, myself included, lucky enough to work with her. Her gentle mindful guidance is woven throughout the pages of this workbook.

Huge thanks to Dr. Jen Gunter, fearless advocate for the truth in women's health and sexuality, for writing the Foreword of this workbook, and for relentlessly debunking women's health myths. I love sharing this space with you!

I am mindful of the fact that I hold a certain privilege that many of my female colleagues and students do not. I am fortunate to hold a Canada Research Chair in Women's Sexual Health, which protects my time and allows me to do the research I do. I also have a supportive family (my kids—Danica, Sebastian, and Luca) and partner (Ed), a home, wonderful friends, and access to the necessities that allow me to thrive in society. I am thankful to my parents, Renato and Germana, and my sisters, Daniela and Sandra, for always believing in me (even when they didn't understand me). I am acutely aware of the number of women who fall through the leaky pipeline in academia and make the difficult decision to leave their university appointments because of a lack of support, both personally and professionally. I do not take this privilege lightly, and I want this workbook to inspire those who face barriers to their professional development to keep going and to seek out trustworthy mentors, which I have been very fortunate to have.

Appendix: What's Next?

HOW TO CONTINUE MINDFULNESS IN YOUR EVERYDAY LIFE

Each chapter of this workbook includes a formal mindfulness practice and asks you to set aside time to do what I call "on the pillow practice." While you did not necessarily sit on a meditation pillow during these practices, they did require you to do some planning to ensure that you had the time, space, privacy, and right context for a longer mindfulness practice. Informal mindfulness practices, in contrast, require no planning or preparation and are ideal ways to bring mindfulness into your everyday life. They are a way of taking the skills you've honed during your formal practice and using them in the regular activities of your day. An analogy to this would be going to the gym and using weights to perform strength exercises (as your formal practice), and then using your strength and agility in your day-to-day life to pick things up and prevent injury (as your informal practice).

Here is a list of informal mindfulness practices that we have recommended as part of our mindful sex groups:

1. **Mindful eating:** Set aside 10 minutes every day to eat mindfully. This means taking a meal, or a portion of a meal, that you planned to eat anyway, and doing so mindfully, eating more slowly and using all of your senses to really experience each bite of the food. You may find yourself eating more mindfully all of the time!

2. **Mindfulness in a regular daily activity:** Choose an activity that you do every day, and bring mindfulness to it—for example, brushing your teeth. You can use all of your sensations to make brushing your teeth a very different experience from what it usually is!

3. **Mindful walking:** Bring mindfulness to walking every day. You might choose particular situations for these mindfulness practices—for example, walking from the parking lot to your office or walking down the aisles of the grocery store.

4. **Mindfulness of sounds:** Bring mindful attention to the sounds that meet your ears throughout the day—for example, while you are washing the dishes, sitting on the bus, or waiting in line. Rather than analyzing the source of the sound, or making sense of the sound itself, simply let all of the sound qualities reach your ears and experience them as they are. You can also do this with music that does not have lyrics.

5. **Mindful standing:** When you are standing in a lineup, instead of reaching for your phone, make it a mindful experience by paying attention to the physical sensations in your feet and legs as you are standing.

6. **Mindfulness of your body:** Take time every day to tune in to your internal physical sensations by doing a brief Body Scan.

7. **Mindfulness during physical affection with a partner:** While you are hugging your partner, holding hands, kissing, lying beside each other while watching a movie, or engaging in any other instance of physical proximity with your partner, try to bring mindful awareness to the points of contact between the two of you.

HOW TO PLAN FOR A LIFETIME OF MINDFUL SEX

You can have a lifetime of mindful sex. Now that you have practiced mindfulness formally, informally, during partnered nonsexual contact, and together with sexual arousal, you have all the building blocks you need to make sex a truly mindful experience.

That said, roadblocks do crop up, so do not feel demoralized if you encounter difficulties as you attempt the exercises in this book. If you can anticipate the roadblocks, however, you may feel better equipped to deal with them when they arise. Some of the women who have participated in our mindfulness groups in the past have told me about various struggles they encountered. My team and I collaborated with the women to find possible ways of overcoming those roadblocks. You may find them helpful.

1. **You find yourself avoiding the mindfulness exercises.** This is common. If this happens to you, explore what is preventing you from doing the exercises. Do you feel guilty about taking time for yourself? Are you worried about being interrupted? Are you discouraged or frustrated with yourself sexually and feel these aspects of yourself are difficult to change? The first step is to break the problem into smaller pieces and try to identify exactly why you are avoiding the exercises. You might be skeptical about the value of the exercises or feel that your problem is too big for them to address. Another way of exploring the avoidance is to focus on the physical sensations and thoughts related to "avoidance."

2. **You feel guilty about taking time for yourself.** Give yourself permission to take this time for yourself. This may be easier to achieve if you are not under pressure to be quick but have chosen a time when you feel good about yourself and your environment.

3. **You are too tired to practice.** Scheduling practice at the end of a busy day when you are exhausted is a sure way to feel resentment toward these exercises. If you are able to vary the times at which you practice, you will have a greater sense of what time of day works best for you. Also, being tired can be a great opportunity to notice sensations of tiredness. How do you know you are tired? What specific physical sensations, thoughts, and so on, are present that make up the experience of "tiredness"? What can you observe about how you relate to "tiredness"? Are the sensations of tiredness constant or do they change over time?

4. **Doing the exercises leaves you feeling bad about yourself and lowers your mood.** How you are feeling about yourself before doing the exercises can affect how you experience them. Immediately before an exercise, take note of what your mood is and what thoughts are present. If you have any negative thoughts or images or bad feelings about yourself or your body, try not to judge yourself for having them.

5. **You have been unable to keep up your practice and feel like you have lost momentum.** You find yourself wondering how to get started again. Remind yourself that you have built up considerable practice during the past several weeks of working through this workbook, and that you have not "lost" or "ruined" your practice just because you lost your momentum for a while. Starting today, you can do something, even if it is just a little. When life seems to be getting in the way and you are struggling to find time to practice, any amount of practice is helpful, even a few minutes. Try to be kind and compassionate to yourself. Remember that ups and downs are normal. You lost the habit of practicing for a time, and that is in the past now. Just focus on the present moment and getting back into a practice.

What other roadblocks do you imagine might crop up? Write about these in your journal.

LOOKING BACK, LOOKING FORWARD

Think back to your original intention when you picked up this workbook. What were you hoping to learn? Where are you now with that goal? Have you reached it? Has your goal changed as a result of bolstering your awareness of incorporating mindfulness into your life (more regularly)? Maybe you have "let go" of a single wish once you realized that it was not realistic. Or maybe, now that you have discovered the power of mindfulness, you wish to bring mindfulness to all aspects of your life.

Regardless of what your original and current goals were/are, I invite you to set an intention about how, where, and when you will bring mindfulness into your life and into your sex life in particular. Will you continue to set aside twenty to thirty minutes a day for a formal mindfulness practice? Will you continue to practice mindfulness informally during a preselected set of activities? Will sensate focus with your partner be something you do regularly, or perhaps it will be something you revisit when you are struggling with your own sexual response or your sexual encounters with a partner, as a way of "resetting"?

In your journal, write down how you intend to bring mindfulness into your life and into your sexuality from today onward. Think back to the struggles and strategies you read about at the end of each chapter. Which struggles do you anticipate encountering as you continue with mindfulness, and what strategies will you use?

IN BETTER SEX THROUGH MINDFULNESS, I wrote: "Satisfying sex is quite simply *not possible* without mindfulness... To be fully present with each sensation, without judgment or commentary, is what I think has been missing from sex for the countless women who are dissatisfied with sex. It cannot be packaged up in a little pink pill. It cannot be injected or placed on the arm in patch form. It is simple but not easy. It requires a lifetime commitment to practice."

My wish for you is this lifetime commitment. My wish for you is mindful sex.

References

Blue, V. *Best Women's Erotica*. Cleis Press, 2007–2015.

Bright, S. *Herotica: A Collection of Women's Erotic Fiction*. Fireweed, Inc., 1998.

Dubberley, E. *Garden of Desires: The Evolution of Women's Sexual Fantasies*. Ebury Publishing, 2013.

Heiman, J. R., and J. LoPiccolo. *Becoming Orgasmic: A Sexual Growth Program for Women*. Prentice Hall Press, 1976.

Herbenick, D., E. Bartelt, T. C. Fu, B. Paul, R. Gradus, J. Bauer, and R. Jones. "Feeling Scared During Sex: Findings from a US Probability Sample of Women and Men Ages 14 to 60." *Journal of Sex & Marital Therapy* 45, no. 5 (2019): 424–439.

Herbenick, D., M. Reece, S. Sanders, B. Dodge, A. Ghassemi, and J. D. Fortenberry. "Prevalence and Characteristics of Vibrator Use by Women in the United States: Results from a Nationally Representative Study." *Journal of Sexual Medicine* 6 (2009): 1857–1866.

Kabat-Zinn, J. *Full Catastrophe Living: Using the Wisdom of Your Body and Mind to Face Stress, Pain, and Illness*. Random House, Inc., 1990.

Lehmiller, J. J. *Tell Me What You Want*. Da Capo Press, 2018.

Lehmiller, J. J., J. R. Garcia, A. N. Gesselman, and K. P. Mark. "Less Sex, but More Sexual Diversity: Changes in Sexual Behavior during the COVID-19 Coronavirus Pandemic." *Leisure Sciences* 43, no. 1–2 (2021): 295–304.

Meston, C. M., and D. M. Buss. "Why Humans Have Sex." *Archives of Sexual Behavior* 36, no. 4 (2007): 477–507.

Mintz, L. B. *Becoming Cliterate: Why Orgasm Equality Matters—and How to Get It*. HarperOne, 2017.

Mitchell, K. R., C. H. Mercer, G. B. Ploubidis, K. G. Jones, J. Datta, N. Field, et al. "Sexual Function in Britain: Findings from the Third National Survey of Sexual Attitudes and Lifestyles (Natsal-3)." *The Lancet* 382, no. 9907 (2013): 1817–1829.

Rumi, J. *The Essential Rumi*. Translated by Coleman Barks. Castle Books, 1997.

Sex Information & Education Council of Canada. (2019). *Canadian Guidelines for Sexual Health Education*. Toronto, ON. sieccan.org/wp-content/uploads/2021/02/SIECCAN-Canadian-Guidelines-for-Sexual-Health-Education-1.pdf.